I0423248

Intermittent Fasting and Autophagy:

Autophagy and Intermittent Fasting for a Healthy Life. How Autophagy and Fasting Could Change Your Life and Heal Your Body. Combine Autophagy and Diet to Burn and Lose Pounds.

© Copyright 2019 by
_____ - All rights reserved.

This eBook is provided with the sole purpose of providing relevant information on a specific topic for which every reasonable effort has been made to ensure that it is both accurate and reasonable. Nevertheless, by purchasing this eBook you consent to the fact that the author, as well as the publisher, are in no way experts on the topics contained herein, regardless of any claims as such that may be made within. As such, any suggestions or recommendations that are made within are done so purely for entertainment value. It is recommended that you always consult a professional prior to undertaking any of the advice or techniques discussed within.

This is a legally binding declaration that is considered both valid and fair by both the Committee of Publishers Association and the American Bar Association and should be considered as legally binding within the United States.

The reproduction, transmission, and duplication of any of the content found herein, including any specific or extended information will be done as an illegal act regardless of the end form the information ultimately takes. This includes copied versions of the work both physical, digital and audio unless express consent of the Publisher is provided beforehand. Any additional rights reserved.

Furthermore, the information that can be found within the pages described forthwith shall be considered both accurate and truthful when it comes to the recounting of facts. As such, any use, correct or incorrect, of the provided information will render the Publisher free of responsibility as to the actions taken outside of their direct purview. Regardless, there are zero scenarios where the original author or the Publisher can be deemed liable in any fashion for any damages or hardships that may result from any of the information discussed herein.

Additionally, the information in the following pages is intended only for informational purposes and should thus be thought of as universal. As befitting its nature, it is presented without assurance regarding its prolonged validity or interim quality. Trademarks that are mentioned are done without written consent and can in no way be considered an endorsement from the trademark holder.

Table of Contents

Introduction

Hello and congratulations for downloading *Intermittent Fasting and Autophagy*. This eBook has been the fruit of many months of research, so I'm very grateful to you for getting it. Thank you!

In the following chapters, the items discussed will be mostly intermittent fasting and autophagy. You will come to know what these concepts are and which is the link between them. There are probably many books with this topic out there, so thanks again for choosing this one. I hope it contains much useful information and helpful advice and it will be one life-changing purchase.

Chapter 1: Intermittent Fasting

Striving for the ideal body, health, and fitness has always been popular. There have always been trends in the world of dieting and exercise, with some of them even being very reckless and dangerous in the long run. We have all heard frightening or plain unsettling stories of tapeworm diets, abuse of diet pills, laxative abuse, but even when we stop looking at those extreme ends, we will always remain baffled at the mere amount of marketing and products concerning body goals. While looking for the best methods which can help us acquire our desired goals, we have all come across a vast number of suggestions, products, and specialists (or even non-specialists) who claim that they have the secret to our ideal body. But despite all this technology, medicine and science involved, the question remains: What should I eat? How should I eat? How should I exercise? And it all comes down to one big question, which is still on the mind of most people, whether they want to lose weight, gain it or improve their athletic performance and appearance: How can I achieve my body goals?

During your weight loss journey, I'm sure you've felt at your wit's end more than once. You have probably researched a lot of diets, nutrition plans, supplements, etc. before you came across this book. You're probably very disappointed by a lot of them. You don't want to try more things that don't work. You need this one thing which is going to finally work for you and help you transition to a healthier lifestyle and a better you. Weight loss is a very tricky process and -when you have a significant amount of weight to lose- it is also a process which will take you a long time. When you actually reach your weight loss goal, you will want to keep it off, so the plan you're going to follow this time should be sustainable and help you maintain your new healthy lifestyle.

In this ocean of -sometimes very misleading-information, it is often very hard to find what works for every one of us. But why look for new exciting methods when we have wisdom from the past to fall back on? Why rely on expensive treatments and pills when we can achieve our body goals in a natural fashion? In this book, you can learn a lot about intermittent fasting, the models you can use to incorporate it in your lifestyle and the way to activate autophagy and come closer to your body goals. About autophagy, I will provide extensive information in chapter 2, but for now, just keep in mind, it is the process your body follows to remove damaged cells, replace them with new ones and in general keep you functioning in a good healthy condition. Here you can also find the scientific explanation of why intermittent fasting works and the relationship between intermittent fasting and autophagy and how you can take advantage of it. So, bear with me and discover the amazing properties of intermittent fasting and how you can use it to improve your own body, mood, and lifestyle. Remember, it's not only about how we look, but also about how we feel. A plan which does not make you feel well is most likely not a sustainable plan for you. On the contrary, if your plan is making you feel deprived and unhappy, it's a distinct possibility that you won't be able to keep it up and even if you reach your weight loss goals, keeping the weight off will be a very hard process. This is the reason why you need to find smart and effective choices, which can work for you and be sustainable.

Lately, more and more people who have tried for years to diet their way to a better lifestyle and a healthier body have made a very sad and shocking discovery. Diets don't work. Of course, they may work in the short run, but their results are most likely not sustainable. And the worst part is, you only find out about that when you have already spent a lot of time, effort and hard-earned money on the latest diet. Diets complicate life, fasting simplifies it. Diets tend to be expensive, fasting is free. Dieting takes time from your life (for preparation and other activities), fasting saves time (less food means less preparation, less shopping, less cleaning). Dieting usually requires specific places (to find a specific meal), fasting is available anywhere, anytime. Diets have variable efficacy; fasting has unquestionable effectiveness. There isn't a more powerful method for reducing insulin and managing body weight than abstaining from food for some time during the day. Is this information something of the present day? Not at all. Even if they did not have the knowledge to support their claims scientifically, many of the ancient cultures of the world already knew the benefits of fasting thousands of years ago. Does fasting mean hunger? Absolutely not! Is your body going to get into starvation mode and your metabolism assuming a snail's pace because of fasting? Not at all.

So as you have understood by now, this book is your beginner's guide to intermittent fasting, achieving autophagy and boosting your fat loss. If you are interested in transforming your eating habits and unlocking all the health benefits you can get by following a process which does not cost you but the price of this book, you are at the right place and the right time. I'm sure by now you are already wondering, is intermittent fasting the way to transform your eating plan and your lifestyle? It could be. Intermittent fasting is not a diet. It doesn't tell you what to eat, but when to eat. Combined with a good nutrition plan for your personal goals and your usual exercise routine, it can boost your immune system, assist your fat loss, help you be more energetic and focused, reduce inflammation, and much more. Sounds interesting? Without further ado, let's venture into the world of intermittent fasting and discover its amazing properties.

Intermittent fasting is a relatively new trend, but it is not at all a new practice. Most of the people who have been on a diet or even researched on dieting information have come across suggestions like not eating after 6 pm. Most of us have skipped breakfast more than once and had lunch as our first meal of the day. Practices like that can constitute intermittent fasting and we have been following them way before this new fancy term came to play. Intermittent fasting is not something for the dieting and exercise elite. On the contrary, for most people, it can prove to be a very manageable way of eating which is also very effective and not costly at all compared to other lifestyle changes.

The presence of the word "fasting" should not be confused with starvation. Starvation refers to the involuntary absence of food and -apart from cases of various eating disorders- is not controlled by the individual. Fasting, on the other hand, refers to abstaining from eating voluntarily, for spiritual or health reasons. And in fact, fasting is something people do every single day. The first meal of the day is called "breakfast" exactly because it breaks the fast which starts after the last meal of the previous night and goes on while we sleep. So, does that mean you have been fasting in your entire life? Yes, you have. Intermittent fasting is a practice based on withholding food for a specific time frame within the day and eating within a smaller time frame - your "eating window" in intermittent fasting terms. There are many different models of intermittent fasting, some easier and some more edgy, so there is a vast amount of methods to choose from within the intermittent fasting spectrum.

Fasting as a key to improving one's health is not a new idea either. Hippocrates, the ancient Greek physician from the island of Kos, who is considered to have written the first medicine book of the western world, was an advocate of fasting for health reasons. It is said that the world-renowned philosophers Plato and Aristotle would also fast for health reasons. The ancient Greeks believed that the observation of nature could help reach helpful conclusions about human health. Hippocrates among others had observed that when animals were sick, they did not have much of an appetite and that this is what happens with most humans too. Hippocrates believed that when one is sick, they should follow their natural tendency not to eat, as "eating while sick is like feeding your illness". But fighting against illness was not the only positive result of fasting to the Greeks. They believed that fasting could make someone more energetic and concentrated. Imagine yourself after a big meal. You might be feeling satisfied, but your body needs to contribute a lot of energy to digest that food. That leads way more blood to the digestive system and there is less left for the brain. That is the reason why we often feel sleepy or tired after a satiating meal. Even a light lunch is sometimes enough to make us feel sleepy and less productive during the next couple of hours.

Fasting is also present in many religions of the world, as it is considered a way of cleansing the body and the mind and learning to say no to temptation. The Muslim way of fasting during the Ramadan period consists of a voluntary withholding of food from sunrise to sunset. The Greek Orthodox fasting (lent) does not have an eating window, but it does limit the types of food one can eat during those days. Fasting as a spiritual process is correlated with purification and resisting temptation, but this notion probably originates by the views of people of those times about the beneficial properties of fasting for the human body. Fasting for any reason, spiritual, health or other, is bound to test your discipline and your self-control.

Intermittent fasting might sound strange to someone who has always known the 5-6 meals a day theory which was prevalent during the past years. Most of us are already familiar with the notion that less than 5 meals a day can slow down your metabolism. And then comes the dreaded starvation mode, which allegedly will make your body consume far less energy, therefore keeping you from losing weight. This has not been scientifically proven. In fact, a survey which was conducted in two groups, of which the first one had 6 meals a day and the other one had 3, with an equal number of calories and nutritional values divided between those meals, showed no significant difference between the two groups. Apart from that, meal planning and prepping for 6 meals a day is exhausting and very time-consuming, especially when it comes to people with a busy lifestyle. The idea behind the theory is actually understandable. Since the body needs energy to digest, 6 meals should take more energy than 3. But if the number of calories and nutritional values is identical, there is no reason to have 6 instead of 3 meals. Most people who have been on traditional diets are growing tired of the relentless meal prepping and grazing they have to perform all day. An unsustainable diet plan is a recipe for failure when one wants to achieve and maintain a healthier body. And eating 6 times a day might be a trigger for people who overeat to feed their habit 6 times a day. We do not want that, now do we?

Another theory which proclaims breakfast the most important meal of the day is much more beneficial to your local bakery and the various snack manufacturers than to your body. The benefits of a good night's sleep and the energy and concentration which follow in the morning are well known for years and even evident in language. "I'll sleep on that" we tend to say about a hard problem which requires us to come up with a solution. And it really does happen that after a good sleep the answer we had been looking for just pops up. This is exactly the level of concentration you have in the morning, after what has been an 8-10 hour fast, if we suppose that one has 8 hours of sleep and does not snack for at least 2 hours before going to bed. Having breakfast is very likely to mean that a good part of that energy will go to digesting it and you will lose that clarity and level of focus. That is not supposed to mean that having breakfast is bad for you. It all comes down to what works for your lifestyle. The point is that many of those misconceptions might hinder your progress, therefore it's good to free oneself from those.

So, is fasting the new breakthrough of dieting? Well, apparently not. People have known and used the advantages of fasting for many years. Why then do we need to look for new and promising revolutionary methods when we already have some wisdom from the past which we can utilize to fulfill our health goals? Intermittent fasting is the process of voluntarily going without food for extended periods of time. It is not a diet but a change in lifestyle. There are many ways to follow that lifestyle and very convincing scientific explanations on why this system can work miracles for your body and health and facilitate your fat loss and other health goals. Intermittent fasting is not a magic pill, it is probably not for everyone and it could match or not match your lifestyle. It is not a diet, but more like a useful tool which you can use to enhance your effort towards your body goals. This book will teach you all you need to know about how to use this tool.

IF How-To

You might already be interested in intermittent fasting but wondering how to do it. How long should you fast? Should you fast completely? Which pattern works best for your own needs? Thankfully there is no one size fits all as far as IF is concerned. There are many intermittent fasting protocols to choose from based on which one better suits your own lifestyle and goals and more and more of them are created every single day.

There are more than sufficient resources online where you can research about IF models and decide which could better work for you. However, as this book is supposed to be your beginner's guide, I have included quite a lot of the most well-known methods for you to see and compare. Let's take a look at a few of those, their strengths and weaknesses and whether you should follow them!

16/8

The 16/8 program is according to many the best way to start your IF journey. 16/8 means that you fast for 16 hours and have an 8-hour eating window. While it can be challenging at first, it is considered to be the easiest beginner plan which will actually be effective. Some people ask whether a 12 hour or 14-hour fast will give them the health benefits of intermittent fasting, but 16 hours seem to make more sense, as the body needs some time to transition between burning glucose to burning fat. This time frame is not identical for everyone. Some people can reach that stage in 6 - 8 hours while others may take up to 12. That means that if you're one of the latter, a fast of 12 hours is absolutely meaningless, while 14 hours will only give you 2 hours left of valuable fat burning.

Pros: Manageable for beginners, can keep up with the usual lifestyle.
Cons: Could seem very basic to more experienced IF followers.

Should I get on the 16/8 plan? It is certainly the easiest start for someone who wants to experiment with IF. This plan is very manageable and someone who already skips breakfast shouldn't find it that hard to follow, to begin with.

You will ask now, what if I fast for 18 or 20 hours?

The Warrior Diet

The name can be misleading, as it is not actually a diet but a way of eating, like all the intermittent fasting methods. They don't tell you what to eat but when to eat it. The warrior diet is based on the way ancient soldiers would feed themselves in times of war. You can picture a march going on from sunrise to sunset, during which they would eat nuts, dried fruit and other snacks rich in energy and nutrients, and then when the sun went down, the warriors would rest and have a quite large amount of food, which was necessary to sustain their energy needs. This is the way of eating on the warrior diet. There is a 20-hour period which is called a fasting period, but in fact, it is an undereating period, as dieters are encouraged to consume apart from non-caloric liquids fruit, vegetables, and hard-boiled eggs. During the 4-hour eating window, dieters are allowed to overeat. This plan can be hard to follow effectively for people who have disordered eating conditions, such as binging and emotional eating, as you still need a caloric deficit and the 4-hour overeating period can send you over your allowance. However, we should mention that the warrior diet suggests organic and healthy choices and avoiding processed foods. The bottom line is, it is a 20/4 plan with some fasting elements, but instead of no eating followed by eating, you have an undereating/overeating period.

Pros: No real "fasting" period, encourages healthy eating choices.
Cons: Possibly hard to keep up with, could be inconvenient to people who do not tend to eat a lot at night.

Should I follow the Warrior Diet? Here we certainly have more difficulty to follow a pattern than the 16/8 plan, but since during the 20-hour fast you can actually consume some products, it could be good for people with very busy lifestyles who are on the move a lot. If you do follow it, make sure to go for healthy choices, as a 4-hour window of "overeating", as it is called in the warrior diet shouldn't become a 4-hour window of poor nutritional choices.

OMAD (One meal a day)

Some consider OMAD to be a stricter version of the warrior diet. The instructions are literally all quite clear, you will be having one meal each day. Most dieters who follow this plan will rely on non-caloric drinks for the fasting period and then consume a big amount of food during their one and only meal of the day. While OMAD can be hard to stick to at first, gradually it becomes easier and it can assist you while cutting on your calorie intake. It is a demanding plan, but taking all of your caloric allowances at once will leave you feeling very satiated after your one meal. Meanwhile, this method can be very helpful to people with a very busy lifestyle, as you will only need to meal prep for one - though quite big- meal per day.

Pros: Good for weight loss, reduced chance of overeating, minimal meal planning.
Cons: Hard for beginners, almost 23-hour fasting periods, could be challenging with social events or outings.

Should I do OMAD? This model can be hard to follow if you are used to eating more than 3 meals a day. It will require significant willpower, as you are only allowed to eat once, but this one meal will be very satiating. It is probably effective for people with very busy lifestyles who find it easier to eat when they get home. It is also a way to ensure you won't end up consuming more calories than your allowance, as with mindful eating, one meal will most likely not give you the chance to overeat. However, it is the only meal you can get through in a day, so you might find yourself having to decline outings which include eating. Though to some, this could be a deterring factor from having oversized restaurant portions, so choose what works for you. What is encouraging to one can be disheartening to someone else and it is important that you can strike the balance for your own weight loss journey.

"Eat-Stop-Eat"

This method features two 24-hour fasting periods in a week. Are you already feeling hungry? Well, it can be tricky to follow, but it is an effective method to keep your caloric intake under control. Dieters are encouraged to eat normally on their 5 eating days, but also make healthy choices. The idea is that by eating normally for 5 days and having no food at all (or in other versions of the method, 500-700 calories) for the remaining 2 days your weekly consumed calories will be significantly less. This, however, does mean you have to be mindful about your eating choices and not overeat on the 5 days. Some people even choose to spread their 24-hour fasting period into 2 days. For example, Ms. A. has her dinner at 6 pm on Monday and stops eating until Tuesday at 6 pm, when she can have dinner, therefore the fasting is not as hard to follow as an 8 am to 8 am 24-hour fast would be.

Pros: 5 days of eating at maintenance, not feeling deprived.
Cons: 2 days of no or minimum calorie intake, maybe not for people with very active lifestyles.

Should I follow the Eat - Stop - Eat model?
Some people find this model to be very sustainable in the long run, because they manage to accommodate their own energy needs with it. For

example, some prefer to eat for the 5 most active days of the week and then live on less or no calories for the 2 days with a milder schedule. However, this method is not a very good way to start with intermittent fasting, as a 24-hour fast when you have never fasted for a long period of time before could make you feel weak and quit fasting altogether.

These are only a few of the most popular choices you have while intermittent fasting. New eating methods are being created every day following an IF related pattern, so you can choose the one that works for you. However, make sure to note that intermittent fasting will not help you lose weight unless you maintain a caloric deficit. It is a common misconception that during the eating window one can eat whatever they want and still lose weight. Of course, this is not the case. Intermittent fasting can have a lot of benefits for your body, but to achieve weight loss you will have to combine it with a healthy diet. However, intermittent fasting does make controlling your caloric intake easier, as you will most likely skip breakfast and if you eat your other meals of the day like you normally would and not overeat during your eating window, your caloric intake will naturally be smaller and you will lose weight.

Intermittent fasting is the method of choice for many people around the world, but did you know it is also the go-to eating plan for many celebrities you might even be envying for their body? Beyoncé has admitted to losing 20 pounds in a short time period by using a diet plan featuring intermittent fasting. The superstar would drink a lot of water with lemon juice, cayenne pepper, and maple syrup and have almost no solid food. When she did eat, her choices were vegetables, fish and protein drinks. Of course, this is not a suggestion to follow that nutrition plan. Nicole Kidman does the 16/8 model, choosing to start her 8-hour eating window at 10 am and eat her last meal at 6 pm. Another idol with an admirable body, Jennifer Lopez, fasts for anywhere between 12 and 18 hours every day and when she eats, she goes for healthy, unprocessed food choices. Other stars who swear by the 16/8 plan or variations of that are Kourtney Kardashian, Selena Gomez, and Halle Berry, while Miranda Kerr goes for the 5:2 diet, which is a variation of Eat - Stop - Eat with minimum calories for the two fasting days of the week. So, if these ladies who look so youthful and healthy believe intermittent fasting is good for them, there is no reason why it wouldn't be good for anyone else who wishes to manage their weight and improve their general health. Intermittent fasting as a way to achieve body goals is also a favorite of many famous men, as Hugh Jackman is said to have been on an IF plan in order to get the athletic appearance his role as Wolverine required.

But let's take a look at everyday people who have nothing to do with celebrities and all the added care that superstars can afford for themselves. The example of D.W. (only initials for anonymity purposes) is very enlightening. D had tried a lot of diets, but he always ended up gaining the weight back and it all boiled down to the fact that diets do not work. One good day D and his coworkers decided to go on a weight-loss competition. D had read about intermittent fasting online and decided to give it a shot, opting for the 5:2 plan despite being a beginner to the world of fasting. He lost 50 pounds in 6 months and apart from winning the competition and the 220 dollars that came with the win, he acquired a better lifestyle, which he kept up after the competition. Another example is the one of A.F. A had heard about intermittent fasting quite a lot of times but was hesitant to try it because of all the information she had been given about having a lot of meals every day to avoid starvation mode. A lost her inhibitions about intermittent fasting, tried it and then also lost 60 pounds in a year and managed to keep this weight off. She's now the healthiest and happiest version of herself and I couldn't be more proud of her. An observation many people who perform intermittent fasting have made is that abstention from food is easier than moderation. Imagine yourself eating only a piece of chocolate or only the recommended serving from a chip bag or mozzarella sticks. We would all agree this is quite hard. But if you know your eating window and abstain from all kinds of food for that period of time, you get in the mindset of not eating for certain hours and you can avoid this kind of temptation. Yes, that dreaded doughnut box in the office. The well- known "one didn't hurt anyone" motto. If you can fast your way out of those situations, you might be surprised to find that you are cutting out many excess calories and much mindless eating, which can be detrimental for your weight loss goals.

Many people ask me, which foods or drinks will break my fast? This is quite an area of debate, as even specialists argue about certain products. However, I'll try to be as informative as possible and give you an understanding of the current debate, but this can only be done after the scientific explanation of intermittent fasting, so bear with me and soon you will have all the information you need right in front of you!

I'm sure that by now you are already thinking about whether this method would work for you. The next chapters will provide a discussion on intermittent fasting, its benefits for your health and how you can use it to achieve autophagy. Autophagy? That's a weird word. What is autophagy and how can it help me, you will ask. Actually, autophagy is a process just as natural as fasting. You should always keep in mind that the human body is one of the most perfect machines - if not the most perfect. It has all the built-in features which can help you in your everyday life, just like a very advanced computer. Autophagy is one of those systems, which can be very beneficial to your health. You can find out all about it in the next chapters.

Chapter 2: Autophagy

Autophagy, like oh so many of the words which are used in the field of medicine, comes from the Ancient Greek language, and especially the word αυτοφαγία (pronounced as autophagia), which consists of the words "αυτός (oneself)" και "φάγω (eat)". So this word refers to a process of consuming elements within the body. I don't know if this seems desirable so far, but take my word for it, it is much better than it sounds!

Autophagy is a normal cellular process by which cell survival is promoted in stress conditions. The cells themselves capture and recycle intracellular proteins and organelles under specific conditions in the lysosomes. Through autophagy, the functionality of the organism is maintained. Autophagy prevents the accumulation of toxic substances from cellular waste and substrates are provided in order to maintain proper metabolic function in cases of starvation. The pathway of autophagy is a highly conserved pathway in eukaryotic cells, which has been shown to be induced in adverse conditions. Those conditions are starvation due to the lack of nutrients, hypoxia, oxidative stress, DNA damage as well as other forms of stress.

In other words, autophagy is a part of your homeostasis. Homeostasis might be ringing a bell from middle school biology; it is exactly those mechanisms that help our body maintain its optimal function. Homeostasis is what makes you sweat when it's hot, it's what gets you back in good health when you're sick. It is widely accepted that autophagy is a cellular homeostatic quality control mechanism, as well as that through this mechanism the fragmentation and elimination of damaged organelles, long-lived proteins, and other damaged cells ingredients is being facilitated.

In addition to recycling cellular ingredients, autophagy plays an important role in a variety of physiological and pathological processes, such as adaptive response to starvation, anti-aging, antigens, placental growth, the elimination of intracellular microbes and genetics stability as well as carcinogenicity. Furthermore, it is estimated that deregulation of autophagy is involved in the pathogenesis of a variety of human diseases, such as neurodegenerative disorders, cardiovascular disorders, diseases, and cancer.

Depending on the load transfer mechanism at the lysosomes, there are three main types of autophagy:

1. **micro-autophagy**, that is the direct delivery of the cargo in lysosomes through lysosomal encapsulation membrane
2. **chaperone-mediated autophagy**, (CMA), which is characterized by the introduction to lysosomes of proteins interacting with specialized escape molecules, and macro-carbohydrates,

3. **macro-autophagy**, the mechanism of which is the most studied within the autophagy functions. Here the load is separated into membrane vesicles known as autophagosomes, which are gradually formed due to the combined action of about 15 proteins associated with autophagy-related proteins (ATG). Autophagosomes may contain cytoplasmic material, inactive proteins, organelles such as mitochondria (mitophagia), peroxidases (hyperphagia), lipid droplets (lipophage), as well as ribosomes (ribophagy) and parts of the core (pyrophage).

Recent studies have shown that autophagy plays a dual role in determining the destiny of cells, since under different circumstances it can either function as a survival mechanism of the cell, or to induce a programmed cellular death. In some cases, the activated autophagy mechanism provides cellular protection, possibly through the elimination of dysfunctional organelles and protein and maintaining the energy balance. On the other hand, autophagy is considered as one type of programmed cell death.

Let us notice that there are three types of cell death:

1. Necrosis: It is a non-programmed type of cell death, causes inflammation reaction in

the cells by immunological activation and, then leads the neighboring cells to death.

2. Apoptosis: It is a programmed cellular death of type I and characterized by its concentration chromatin, DNA fragmentation, and formation of apoptotic particles.

3. Excessively activated autophagy: It is a type II programmed cell death, which consists of the elimination of damaged or abnormal cells.

Although autophagy appears to have both cytotoxic and cytoprotective activity depending on conditions, there is no clear experimental data stating that one type of autophagy is different from the other. For example, in the case of cancer cells, depending on the type of volume and the extent of the damage in DNA, autophagy can have both cytoprotective and cytotoxic functions.

By now you must be feeling that there is quite a lot of science going on. Indeed, the term autophagy is very present in medical research, so it is inevitable that some terms will be difficult to grasp. But this is why you have this book in your hands so that these complex notions become very clear for what they can offer to your daily life. An easier way to put it is that autophagy is an organized, smooth process that degrades and recycles cellular components or replaces old cell parts. Autophagy occurs in subcellular organelles, which are destroyed and rebuilt with new ones that are replaced. Old cell membranes, organelles, and other cellular debris are removed by sending them to lysosomes, specific organelles containing enzymes for protein degradation. Autophagy was first described in 1962 when researchers noticed an increase in the number of lysosomes in rat liver cells after glucagon injection. The story begins very early when the father of the autophagous Belgian cytologist Christian de Duve discovers the lysosome (the discovery for which he was awarded the Nobel Prize in 1974) and becomes dad and godfather of this new concept, which is none other than autophagy. The cells, due to their metabolism and the toxic environment, are filled up with harmful substances from which they must escape. Thanks to autophagy, they are released from toxins and self-repaired. The lysosomes contain enzymes capable of breaking down into them and thus form the key organelle for this process, i.e. internal recycling.

Research on autophagy has been getting more and more popular over the recent years, with the 2016 Nobel Prize for Medicine going to Yoshinori Ohsumi for his research on autophagy. The contribution of this scientist to what we know about autophagy today is very important, so we should discuss a few basic elements of his Nobel winning work. Although scientists agreed that this mechanism exists and that lysosomes play a minor role, they were known by the early 1990s when Ohsumi began to study how the cell controls the process of autophagy. His companion is yeast, a single-cell microorganism popular among scientists. As he said in his Nobel interview, "There is no finish line for science. When I find an answer to one question, another question comes up. I have never thought I have solved all the questions. So, I have to keep asking questions about yeast. " Due to its size - the yeast is very small - its organs are almost invisible. No one could, therefore, be sure that autophagy even occurs in these fungi. Ohsumi, therefore, thought he would block the process, see what would happen and let the unnecessary substances accumulate so that the organisms become visible. Knowing that autophagy may be a reaction to starvation began a "strict diet" on fungi. So within a few hours, he noticed that vacuoles were filled and therefore were autophagous vesicles. Not only did it prove the autophagy in the fungi but also found the way it will study it. After this breakthrough, 8,000,000 crowns, that is the equivalent of 830,000 euros and about 930,000 US dollars, will be given to Ohsumi to pursue his research into the discovery of the mechanisms of autophagy. One would ask, why such a huge interest in autophagy? Why did Ohsumi devote all those years and time into studying yeast? Autophagy, therefore, based on its studies and others, helps prevent cancer, maintain metabolism and protect against various diseases. While in cases when autophagy becomes dysfunctional, neurological diseases, diabetes, and malignancies can develop. In Parkinson's disease, for example, the mechanism of autophagy is important for brain nerve cells, where defective proteins can kill cells and cause worsening symptoms, such as tremor. In Parkinson's disease there are problems in removing abnormal proteins, so understanding the mechanism of autophagy helps to find drugs that help in this process, thus limiting the symptoms. The future according to Mr. Ohsumi will be drugs that will intervene in the autophagy process and will regulate it to the benefit of the body. The committee said that "its findings have led to a new ideological structure in understanding how the cell is recycling its content" and stressed that "they have paved the way for understanding many physiological processes such as adaptation to malnutrition or the response to the infection."

So, you do like how this autophagy sounds, right? Stay tuned for more information on how it works and how you can achieve it and enhance its function while it's cleaning up your body and making you healthier. While many detox supplements and diets are being marketed promising that they will help you detox your body and even claiming that they will stimulate your autophagy mechanisms, the truth is way more simple and, thankfully, way less expensive. This book will show you how to avoid products you do not need and reach autophagy with the help of a fully natural method people have been following for thousands of years. You guessed it; this method is fasting!

But before we move on to how you can activate autophagy by fasting, we should definitely answer any doubts you may have about those two terms and their scientific reliability. Cell death might sound a little threatening until you see what the process of autophagy can do for your body. Don't worry, you won't have to look for this information and get tangled in medical journals, as the next chapter will make everything crystal clear for you. Where others use advertising to convince about their methods, I will only need to use good old science.

Chapter 3: The Science Behind

The science behind the two principles we have already examined in this book - autophagy and intermittent fasting - is very encouraging for people who wish to try IF. When it comes to your nutrition plan, your exercise, and your body, nothing should be left to chance. We have all heard the saying "your body is a temple". While this is a notion which points to the fact that we need to keep ourselves healthy and clean, it doesn't capture the essence of the self-love you need to change your habits. What does that have to do with a chapter dedicated to boring science, you may ask. Well, in your process of self-improvement, I trust that you will want your research on the new method you will be following to be as precise as possible and unfortunately the only way to assist you in that is to give you a brave helping of the scientific facts behind the terms which have been discussed.

In order to understand why intermittent fasting works and why it is good for us, we should take a look at what happens to our body when we eat and how we gain, lose, or maintain our weight. When you start eating, the taste buds send pleasure messages to the brain, who in turn requests more food. As you chew, the enzymes present in the saliva break down the sugars and the starch you just consumed. Five minutes later, your stomach is trying to dissolve the food and forward it to the small intestine, from where nutrients such as fat and protein are sent into the circulatory system. If you have had more food than you can handle, the stomach and the small intestine alert the brain through intestinal hormones, such as YY peptide (PYY). You should imagine their message as "We need help". After about half an hour, your blood vessels become less flexible. After dessert, insulin levels have increased in their attempt to control the amount of sugar that flows into your bloodstream. The drowsiness that you feel after the meal comes from your stuffy stomach, which sends a message to the brain. Then your brain recruits all the energy of your body into the hard struggle with a digest. If you have had quite a lot of excess food, your stomach might be causing you discomfort, even pain. About an hour later, the liver has transformed the food into nutrients, which are absorbed by the organs. If you've eaten at maintenance, most fat and calories you've consumed will turn into short-lived energy. If you have eaten more than your maintenance, this excess amount will be stored on your hips, abdomen, and buttocks. About two hours after you have eaten, the stomach is empty again. This process takes a lot of your valuable energy and, if you have been overeating, makes you gain weight. If you are eating fewer calories than your body consumes, you will eventually lose weight.

Weight Loss Chart

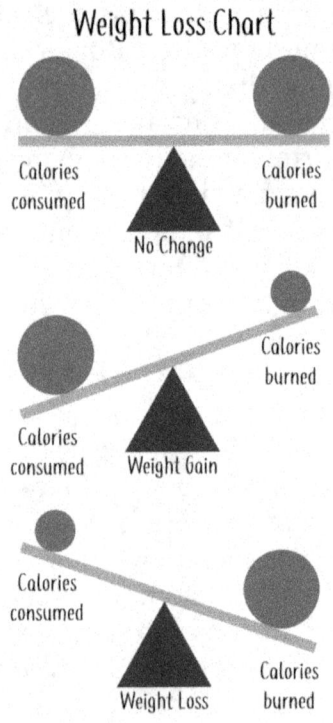

This is exactly what is being explained in this chart. The caloric balance (otherwise, caloric equilibrium) means that there are three possible ways to go: weight gain, weight loss, and maintenance.

In order to lose weight, your calories consumed should be less than your calories burned. This can be achieved by a proper nutrition plan for your needs and exercise. It is quite true that exercising enough to completely cancel a bad diet is very hard and, in most cases, not realistic at all, so the main effort has to come from your eating.

Chart 3.1 - Caloric balance

Maintenance is achieved when you eat as many calories as your body needs to sustain itself. You won't gain or lose any weight. This is usually the stage where things go wrong when you have to keep the weight off after a weight loss journey. This is why at this stage it is very important that you have learned the skills and the mechanisms which will help you keep your new body in top shape.

If your calories burned are less than your calories consumed, you are going to gain weight. If you have a weight gain goal, this is exactly what you want. However, if you find out that you are gaining weight while you don't wish to gain any, you have to revisit your food choices and find out what is to blame. There are some genetics, hormonal and other factors which can definitely influence weight loss, but the main cause you are gaining is in your eating.

Many overweight people think they are not eating that much, while in fact, they might be consuming hundreds of calories over their maintenance. Similarly, many people who wish to gain weight might be feeling that they are eating too much food to actually not gain. This happens because our perception of food is always based on what we are used to rather than our knowledge of the nutrients and energy we get vs the ones we need. This is why it is important to monitor what you eat. If you think your weight gain or loss is not justifiable based on your eating habits, try recording what you are eating in a week and then making the necessary adjustments.

About Intermittent Fasting (and Fasting in General)

Food is very enjoyable to most if not all people. It is there at our social outings, it is there at the Sunday family table. We all have memories of recipes, smells, dinners with friends and family. But the bottom line is, if we are serious about our health goals, we should separate this function of food from the one our body is concerned about. We eat to fuel our body and give it the energy to get us through our daily activities. But what exactly happens when we fast and why is it so beneficial?

Our body has two main sources of energy. Glucose and fat. While we want to get rid of our dreaded fat deposits, the body tends to get lazy and go for the easier solution. When glucose is available, it is what will be consumed first. This means that if we are grazing on carbohydrates all day long, we don't give our body the chance to burn body fat, as there is always glucose available. However, if the body finds out that there is no more glucose, it has no choice but to burn fat. This is exactly what we want to achieve by intermittent fasting. Other diets and eating models, such as the keto diet are also based on the transition between a fed and a fasted state. We have to remember that the body is programmed to withstand periods of low food availability. We are currently experiencing a lifestyle which guarantees that we can be having food every day, even multiple times in a day. But things haven't always been this way. In the early days of human evolution, people couldn't know how far away in time their next meal would be. Therefore, our body has developed many mechanisms to keep functioning in situations of limited food availability.

To be more specific, there are five stages in the transition between a fed and a fasted state. You can see them in the table below, but I will also explain them to you.

Stage 1: The fed state, right after your meal. The glucose is exogenous (a fancy Greek word which suggests that it's coming from the outside) because you are consuming it at that moment. Insulin levels at this stage are high and the glucose is being stored at all tissues to be used later. Excess glucose is stored as glycogen in the liver.

Stage 2: The post-absorptive phase, the one you will mostly utilize during your intermittent fasting along with Stage 3. Within the first 6-24 hours of fasting, the body has no more spare glucose, insulin levels fall and the body starts breaking down glycogen for energy.

Stage 3: When you make it to this stage, the body is running low on glycogen. The liver needs to create new glucose (hence the name, gluconeogenesis, Greek for "creation of new glucose"). And the main ingredient to create new glucose is amino acids. The

Stage 4: This is the stage you have heard people refer to as ketosis. The body enters lipolysis, breaking down fat for energy. Fatty acids are used for energy by the entire body, except for the brain. Your brain tissues are being fueled by ketone bodies, which increase dramatically during fasting. People on keto often speak of better concentration and focus.

Stage 5: Protein conservation phase: In this stage, your body has high levels of growth hormone, which means that it can maintain muscle mass and lean tissues. The energy which is necessary for the maintenance of your basal metabolism is almost entirely met by the use of free fatty acids and ketones. Increased adrenalin prevents the decrease in metabolic rate.

Stage	I	II	III	IV	V
Origin of blood glucose	Exogenous	Glycogen, Hepatic gluconeogenesis	Hepatic gluconeogenesis, glycogen	Gluconeogenesis, hepatic and renal	Gluconeogenesis, hepatic and renal
Tissues burning glucose	All	All except liver. Muscle at diminished rates.	All except liver, muscle and adipose tissue at diminished rates.	Brain, RBCs, renal modulia, a small amount by muscle	The brain at a diminished rate, RBCs, renal medulla
Major brain fuel	Glucose	Glucose	Glucose	Glucose, ketone bodies	Ketone bodies, glucose

Chart 3.2 - Fed to fasted state phases

While intermittent fasting will not utilize all those stages, you can certainly combine it with the keto diet, as many people do. However, intermittent fasting can be useful without keto as well. In this table, you can see that in no stage does your body break down muscle mass. In order for this to happen, your body would have to run out of fat, something which is very highly unlikely with our way of living.

If this interesting but also highly theoretical science explanation is not your cup of tea, let's skip to the point where intermittent fasting assists in weight loss. As it is an area where much research has been conducted, especially in recent years, there are results to suggest that intermittent fasting does indeed assist in weight and fat loss. It is important to remember that those two are not the same thing and intermittent fasting is a process which can help anyone on their weight loss journey to not end up as a "skinny fat" person. With intermittent fasting, you can lower your fat percentage while losing weight, which is a very nice added benefit, considering the number of people who reach their weight loss goals only to find that their body fat -- or at least quite some of it -- is right where they left it. As the following graph shows, as the hours you are fasting increase, so increases your fat burning.

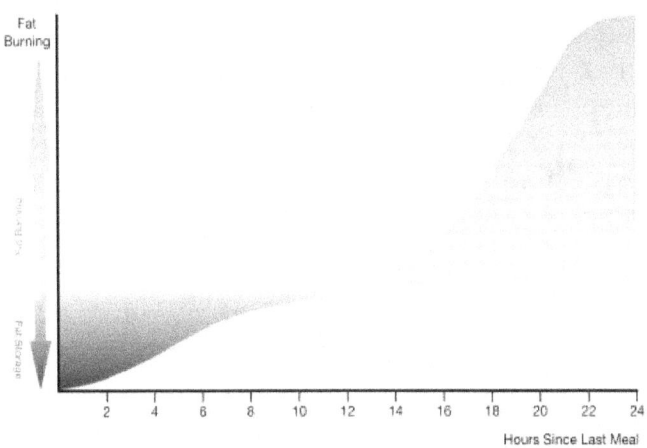

Fat Burning During Fasting

Hours Since Last Meal

Chart 3.3 - Fat burning during a 24-hour fast.

What you will immediately notice about the information this graph conveys is that when you move past about 10 hours of fasting, your fat storage is inactive while your fat burning is starting to increase. As you can see, a 24-hour fast is very effective, but even the 16/8 plan can give you a few good hours of fat burning every single day. There is a very interesting analogy comparing our stored fat with a bank, while glucose is like the wallet we carry. Just like when we are out of money in our wallet, we take some from our bank, when our body is done processing glucose for energy, it turns to the stored fat. This is exactly what we want and it's also an interesting allegory.

As you can see in the following chart, intermittent fasting is a great way to boost your human growth hormone. This peptide hormone is responsible for growth, cell reproduction, and regeneration and in general, human development. This hormone is something people who work out and want to enhance their athletic appearance really want to boost, this is why so many of them are already on intermittent fasting plans. Let's take a look at the science.

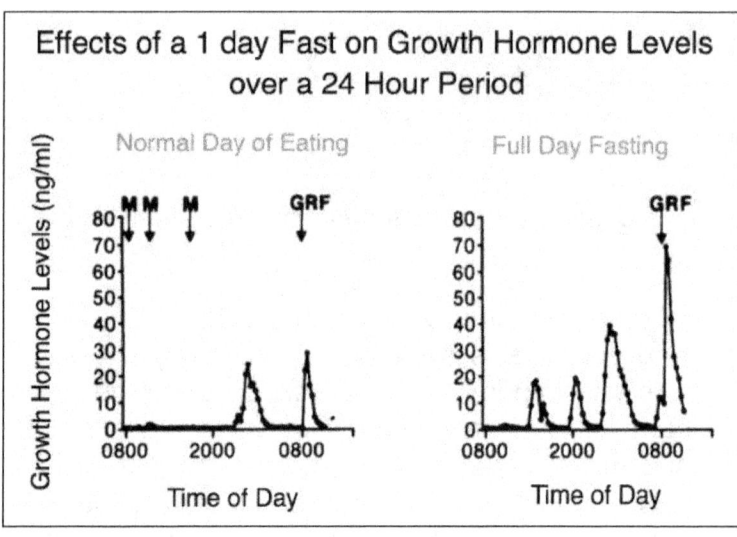

Chart 3.4 - Human Growth Hormone (HGH) during a 24-hour fast.

The graph is showing us the difference between eating normally and fasting for a full day as far as HGH is concerned. While most intermittent fasting plans will not have you fasting for 24 hours, it is certainly an option. Fewer hours of fasting will still have a positive effect on HGH levels in your body. Human growth hormone does many beneficial things for your body, but just allow me to discuss that in the chapter where I'll tell you all about the benefits of intermittent fasting.

I do hope the scientific explanation of intermittent fasting is clear enough by now and has not drained you of your energy and determination to keep reading. In the next paragraph, you can see some scientific facts about autophagy.

About Autophagy

So, as we have already seen, autophagy is apart from a fancy Greek word a very useful procedure for your body. It is a crucial part of your homeostasis, the mechanisms which make sure to keep you in top function and repair any damage that might occur to you due to the environment, and this means you want to keep it functioning well.

As we mentioned earlier, autophagy is a process in which the body does away with all the harmful substances or cells and prevents a number of diseases. As one can see in this informative picture, autophagy slows down aging, fights infection, reduces the chances of Type 2 diabetes, is responsible for the prevention of quite a few diseases and it manages cell death and changes within the structure of the cells to achieve these goals.

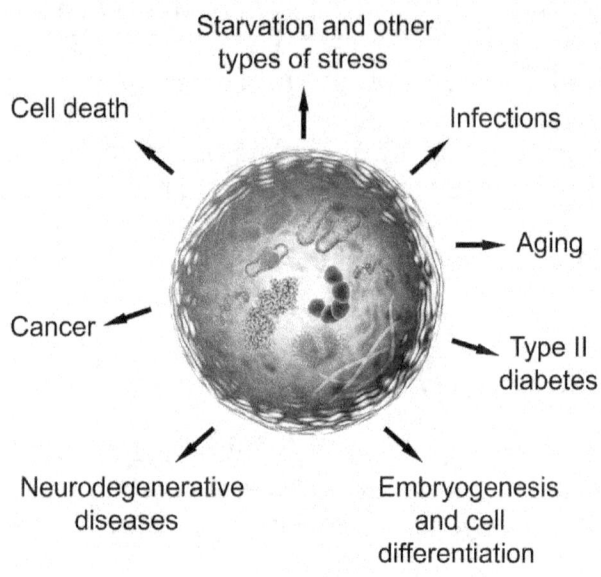

Chart 3.5 - Autophagy functions

The contribution of autophagy to cellular health contains important physiological and pathological roles for this closely monitored procedure. Indeed, autophagy has been found to be of crucial importance during the development of mammals. In addition, recent research has found that autophagy is a critical factor which keeps us safe against a wide range of diseases and disorders. But why exactly do we research on autophagy? Examining the participation of autophagy in development and disease is vital to a fuller understanding the function of it and the implications which may arise while maintaining health or treating illnesses. Although we can by now partially understand its overall morphology and function, information about different steps is emerging in this complex course. During the process, many catabolic pathways within the cell break down large molecules. In particular, conjugation of a small protein called ubiquitin to another cellular protein - often followed by the consequent addition of ubiquitin molecules to create a chain - can label this protein fit for degradation by the proteasome, resulting in amino acid release. A very similar breaking down process takes place as far as carbohydrates and lipids are concerned too.

So, why is autophagy so unique and why worth all this research? The answer is to be found in the flexibility of the size of the autophagosome and the choice of the cargo. Autophagy can promote mass degradation for a large number and variety of substrates, allowing cells to quickly and efficiently produce recycled basic building materials in view of a wide range of nutritional deficiencies. In addition, autophagy is the only function in the body which is able to break down entire organelles within the cell, either randomly or in a targeted manner - a critical process for maintaining homeostasis in the complex landscape of the eukaryotic cell. The central metabolic sensor of the cell, the TOR1 complex (TORC1 or MTORC1 in mammals), is susceptible to the availability of amino acids and growth factors and inhibits the induction of autophagy when these components are abundant. When the cells starve from these molecules, TORC1 / MTORC1 is inactivated, promoting an increase in autophagy. This does mean that autophagy is activated during a lack of energy, which will bring us to chapter 4 and how you can activate it through intermittent fasting. Meanwhile, other molecular regulators control cells for the condition of various nutrients, such as glucose or energy in the form of ATP, and cause autophagy when such nutrients or metabolites reach critically low levels.

Once autophagy begins, it is regulated by many proteins related to autophagy (in general called ATG. These proteins work together to coordinate the formation of the phagophore and the subsequent stages of autophagy. The yeast ATG genes were discovered in the 1990s by Dr. Ohshumi, transforming autophagous research, which was largely descriptive, in a highly mechanistic and molecular level. The experiments using the genetically trappable Saccharomyces cerevisiae incubator dough have played an important role in helping scientists decipher the basic mechanisms behind autophagy. Research into other organisms followed shortly, revealing remarkable evolutionary conservation in nature and the operation of autopsy machines from dough to man.

While I do imagine that this might be your least favorite chapter, as there is quite a lot of biology involved and you might feel like high school has started all over again, it is indeed important to know how autophagy works. The following graph shows us exactly that for every step of the process.

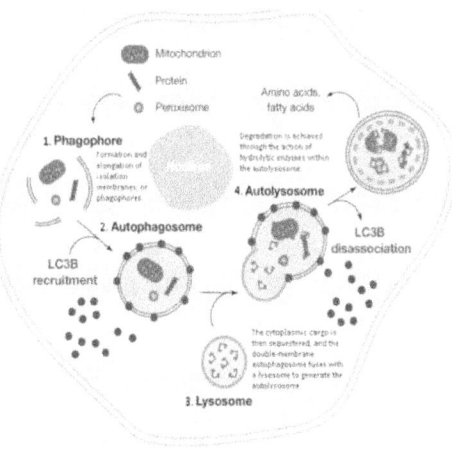

Chart 3.6 - Autophagy in steps

While the whole process of autophagy is now somewhat clear to scientists and certainly much more understandable than it was in the 1990s, when the first pioneering researches were conducted, the field is still tough at work trying to find and fit into many pieces missing from the puzzle. The donor of the membrane for the autophagous, for example, has not been specifically documented. Similarly, we do not fully understand how phagorop extension is regulated or what dictates the frequency of the autophagous generation. Yet more questions arise when we consider that many types of autophagy are highly selective and the initiation and regulation of these processes remain mysterious. Further understanding of these selective pathways is vital because it is closely linked to fetal development, healthy development, growth and prevention of human disorders.

If one had to explain autophagy with the simplest words possible, it would literally be the caregiver of your body. Autophagy is the process which will be activated if something is wrong with you on a cellular level and will not stop until the threat is long gone. Based on that, it is understandable that we want to boost our autophagy and use it to the best of our advantage. Which happens to be exactly what you will read about in the next chapter, so stay tuned.

Chapter 4: Intermittent Fasting and Autophagy

As you probably have guessed by now, intermittent fasting is your way to activating autophagy. The good news is, you can train your body towards autophagy and make this process function even better for you. You never thought you would be asking about how to best eat yourself, now would you? In fact, autophagy is the most beneficial self-cannibalization you are going to encounter and there are a few ways to activate it through diet and exercise. Training your body to eat itself is something you will never regret doing. While we haven't yet discussed the benefits this process has for you, I am sure you're already interested in this absolutely natural process. How many supplements and diets claim they can help us detox ourselves, get rid of unnecessary substances and improve our performance? In fact, the human body is perfectly capable of detoxing itself and does not need any supplements in order to achieve this. The only thing you need is to pay attention to how you can activate autophagy in a natural and sustainable way. While intermittent fasting is not the only way to do so, we believe it is the most efficient way.

Intermittent fasting is always associated with autophagy, with many types of research over the last decade suggesting a positive correlation between those two and longevity or preventing diseases. It has been found that intermittent fasting and autophagy can make the body fight against cancer more effectively and enhance the treatment procedure for people going through chemotherapy. So, if we recall all the science related to autophagy, we definitely remember that it is triggered by a stress factor. So, if we want it to be activated, we have to invent a stress factor. Fasting seems to have the solution right at hand. Researchers are attempting to find out once and for all why fasting is joined to longevity for years. Science laboratory mice and monkeys that participate in lab studies tend to have a longer life than their often-fed peers.

Research finds that taking fewer calories or fasting for a good part of the day actually activates genes that tell cells to preserve resources. The cells get in a preservation or "famine mode," wherever they are, remarkably, way more immune to malady or cellular stress. They conjointly enter the stage we earlier called as autophagy, in which the body begins to wash out the recent, unwanted, and gratuitous cellular material, likewise as someone would be fixing and recycling broken elements to keep a machine in good function. In one study, mice that fasted for twenty-four hours showed high numbers of autophagosomes, the signs that autophagy is functioning. Now, we've to use caution linking this on to humans as a result of mouse metabolism is far quicker than ours. Whereas autophagy is incredibly troublesome to live outside of a science laboratory atmosphere, several specialists agree that the autophagy method initiates in humans once 18-20 hours of fast, with supreme advantages occurring once the 48–72-hour mark has been reached. If this sounds discouraging, detain mind that doing intermittent fasts can still provide you with advantages, however sporadically (a few times a year betting on your personal risk factors) you would possibly contemplate an extended quick fast to completely activate autophagy and do some spring cleanup for your cells. Of course, you ought to visit your doctor before embarking on any fast regime. The activating of autophagy is considered to be one of the benefits of an intermittent fasting regime. When levels of insulin are high, autophagy can be hindered and not work as good as they can be working. Therefore, an intermittent fasting scheme, which reduces the insulin levels and keeps providing with a stressor can keep your autophagy mechanisms healthy and providing for the rest of your body.

The mechanism of autophagy is triggered when the body is experiencing nutrient depletion. During fasting - not eating, glucagon levels rise, which warns the brain of lack of food, and the latter receives a series of countermeasures to cope with the sudden "risk". It is an ancient mechanism. Thousands of years ago, food was not given, and therefore we have developed special ways of dealing with such situations. In this case, the brain activates the process of autophagy. And because nothing happens accidentally, the body begins with the breakdown of old cells, inflammations, and bacteria. It begins to decompose the accumulated "garbage" caused by simple diseases to what we call aging. Yes, rightly read, fasting in addition to triggering autophagy stimulates growth hormone, which has anti-aging action. Therefore, fasting can reverse the process of aging, releasing our body from old cellular garbage and replacing it with new parts. Thus, autophagy is a natural, smooth process that is carried out in a controlled manner and helps to renew our body and fight many diseases, including inflammatory diseases, infections, cancer, and Alzheimer's disease.

But how do we know that fasting activates autophagy? It has been proven in many research attempts, but we can also be relatively sure about it on a theoretical level. Both carbohydrates and proteins increase insulin and reduce glucagon, the substance that activates the process of autophagy. This is why a large number of nutritionists now support partial fasting, the process whereby the body remains foodless for several hours, either in the afternoon or in the morning of each day. There are counter-arguments to this methodology, but the bottom line is that fasting, be it a religious practice or a dietary practice can have significant health benefits. Of course, we always have to keep in mind that balance is everything. Excessive autophagy can be devastating. Because, after the decomposition of the "rubbish", there might be problems with your muscle tissue. So, if you are healthy, you can follow mild forms of fasting. However, if you suffer from a condition and you want to have a fasting treatment, then it should be done under the supervision of a specialist.

However, do not worry, as the next chapter of this book will explain to you exactly how to avoid excessive autophagy and keep on the levels you need for your body to be on its best performance. Short term fasting, such as intermittent fasting, has been proven to increase neuronic autophagy at a very satisfactory level.

It has also been found that religious fasts are positively correlated to this process, with many scientists going back to these thousand-year-old practices and examining them for their health benefits. A very interesting research was done on the Orthodox monastic fasts and their effects on health combined with the keto diet as a preparatory method. Historically, the role of religious fasting has been imposed in order to improve health because fasting essentially means abstinence from some foods and a few meals in the day. Monastic fasts are made with only two meals a day with a distance of about 12 hours between them, based on vegetables, nuts, seeds, and seafood. This serves the purpose of believers having clarity of mind (brain) to pray (or meditate) by being in a state of ketosis. This apostolic approach to orthodox fasting is beneficial to the body. First, it causes ketosis that significantly reduces hunger and secondly promotes autophagy and molecular mechanisms of repairing damage at the cellular level. So, to do it right, this research showed we should focus on non-starchy vegetables, seafood, avocados, olives, fermented vegetables such as pickles, nuts, and seeds such as almonds, sesame seeds, and tahini. Of course, we must ensure before we start fasting to have high levels of ferritin and vitamin B12. These two nutrients are the only ones that can be reduced during forty days of fasting. In conclusion, this type of religious fasting can be more than healthy as long as certain conditions are met, such as relying mainly on non-starchy vegetables and not on starchy foods and sugars that stimulate insulin and lead to hunger while making the process of orthodox fasting extremely difficult. If one concentrates on vegetables, seafood, avocados, olives, fermented vegetables (sugar-free pickled), nuts, seeds, tahini, coconut milk, Japanese pasta and shirataki rice, and bread-free bread but tahini and coconut flour, the monastic fasting can provide with much of the elements of intermittent fasting and keto. When low-carbohydrate fasting promotes ketosis, you can lose weight, improve your glucose and insulin levels. Ideally, a keto-adaptation period of six weeks can be very helpful in order to have good ferritin and B12 storerooms and a smooth transition to Orthodox fasting.

With intermittent fasting, many people ask about what will break a fast and whether they should try dry fasting, so I will try to answer that as extensively as possible. Let's begin with dry fasting. Since ancient times, it has been believed that a certain amount of dry fasting could be beneficial to combat diseases. For the ones who are not familiar with the term, dry fasting refers to fasting without even drinking water. With dry fasting (complete lack of food and water), the body goes into a "holiday phase" where the digestive system, and in particular the endocrine glands, undergo rest, and the body prepares for the next anabolic phase. The modern lifestyle is characterized by an oversupply of goods, tension, stress, and fatigue. Man is fed with the wrong foods at the wrong time and in the wrong way. Food-related diseases, as well as those related to over-consumption of drugs (antibiotics, antipyretics, cortisone, antihistamines, etc.), pose a lot of problems to the body, burdening our physical and mental health. Modern man has already begun to perceive the great importance of proper nutrition to maintain his health. Fasting as a method of treatment for bodily diseases is known from ancient times. But what about consuming water? It is widely believed that it is beneficial and healthy to drink plenty of liquids, especially water, highlighting the benefits of drinking much water. Supporters of this theory claim that by having a lot of liquids they cleanse the kidneys, detoxify the body, cellulite goes away, belly volume decreases, intestinal function improves, spastic colitis is treated, many other diseases are treated and metabolism improved. This view contradicts a tradition we have from ancient Greek and Byzantine texts. In these, it is advisable not only to stop eating while fasting but also to stop drinking water. For example, we can mention Hippocrates, who recommends, when one is healthy, that water is mitigated and when someone is ill, not given at all. So, we should consider which the right outlook is. The first, which has prevailed since 1960 and the second, the second, which has been in force for more than 2,500 years (since 500 BC)? From the behavior of the animals, we know that when they get sick or injured, they automatically abstain from food and water, rest, and in this way - following their instincts - they are healed. In a recent review, published in the Journal of the American Nephrology Society, there is a lack of scientific evidence demonstrating that drinking a lot of fluids is beneficial. According to the text of the review, there is no scientific study and evidence that the kidneys cleanse, nor that the body detoxifies with drinking a lot of water.

As part of the treatment of illness, we have been trying for the last fifteen years to explore the parameters and the effects of oligopolies and drought on the human body. Observations in many patients have shown that consuming too much fluid retards recovery in infectious diseases, increases allergies, improves kidney function, in the case of colonic kidneys increases pain, worsens spastic colitis, increases body weight, worsens breathing and heart function, destabilizing the autonomic nervous system and increasing cellulite. In an ongoing study in December 2007, with 11 volunteers who underwent a five-day to seven-day drought, we investigated a variety of parameters (such as somatometric, hematological, biochemical, renal, hormonal and immunological) during drought.

The volunteers observed in the above study were in good physical condition until the end of the study, except for a small amount of fatigue. Their psychological status was excellent. It should be noted that the drought appears to have strong antidepressant action. Their weight was reduced by about 1.5 kilos a day, all days. Body perimeters were improved by about 1-1.5 cm each, every day. All patients experienced a significant improvement in breathing, as assessed by changes in chest perimeter and by the determination of blood oxygen saturation. The condition of the bowel improved considerably, as was noted by the reduction in abdominal perimeters, but also by the subjective sensation of the volunteers. Also, the hip perimeter was reduced at a rate of about 1 cm per day, which translates into a rapid improvement in cellulite. This study found a negligible loss of muscle mass. Also, throughout the study, the blood pressure of the subjects remained relatively unchanged.

Regarding kidney function, which is mainly evaluated by creatinine, creatinine clearance and electrolytes (K. Na, Cl), it appears not only that it is not adversely affected but is greatly improved. Urea prices gradually increased to a limited extent over the five-day dry fasting. As this substance is not a harmful toxin, this change is not evaluated negatively. Hormone values have shown that the body goes through drought in a different phase of operation, where other hormones are growing and others are reduced in order to provide energy from the inside and, on the other hand, by resting to cure over-functioning endocrine glands.

This procedure reduces insulin, T3, T4, and TSH increase glucagon, cortisol and growth hormone.

These observations show that the body goes through drought in a "holiday phase" where the endocrine glands are resting-down and the body prepares for the next anabolic phase (building new tissues). Hepatic enzymes (SGPT, γ-GT) remain stable, which means that the liver does not burden, whereas hematocrit and hemoglobin are increased.

Some immunological parameters indicative of the ability of the body's defense system to cope with a variety of threats were also looked into by the study. For example, it was found that peripheral blood lymphocytes had increased proliferation capacity. This can be translated as an increased readiness of the immune system to cope with internal enemies (autoimmune diseases) or external enemies (infections). These observations indicate a potential enhancement of the body's self-healing capacity. Therefore, should one dry fast? Apparently, a short and monitored time of dry fasting might also have a positive effect on your body. However, we would not suggest it as a long-lasting weight-loss method. Remember, you need a nutrition plan which can last you for years, perhaps even for the rest of your life, since losing the weight is only one part of the journey, with the other and more difficult part is keeping the weight off.

So, in case you are not dry fasting and you only want to follow intermittent fasting, let's say the 16/8 protocol, you must definitely be wondering about what you can consume during the fasting period. While most hardcore dieters and intermittent fasting specialists have only one answer to that, and this is "water", there are certain things you can consume, depending on your fasting regime. In more detail:

Water: Of course, water has no calories at all and you can consume it during your fasting. Many people ask about sparkling water. You can also consume sparkling water without breaking your fast. About the various flavored waters, you need to make sure they do not contain any added sugar. The best way to go if you prefer your water flavored is to add a couple of slices of lemon - which technically *is* breaking a fast, but in practice, it is fine.

Tea or coffee: While tea and coffee are within the products which have a very small but existing nonetheless amount of calories, most intermittent fasting experts accept that you can consume them. Coffee should be taken black, without sugar and without a creamer. It might be hard to get used to at first, but it is worth it. If black coffee is a too intense taste for you, maybe you can opt for tea as a daily beverage. Green tea is considered the best for intermittent fasting, but black tea will be okay too, provided that you add no sugar and no milk. Some herbal teas which are infused with fruit are not advised, as they, unfortunately, can break your fasts and fruit contains carbohydrates. Of course, if you are tempted to opt for some iced tea or other packed beverage, you should make sure to check there is no added sugar.

Sweeteners: Many intermittent fasting experts disagree about whether zero or very low-calorie sweeteners will break your fast. Some believe that if there are no calories, it's a "go", while others think that the sweet taste can still stimulate your insulin reaction. It would be safe to assume that anything with 0 or very close to 0 calories is not enough to break your fast, but you don't want to go to anything more caloric than that, as it might be healthier than sugar, but your insulin doesn't know that.

Soda: I guess I shouldn't have to stress this, but anything with sugar is out of the question. Some drink soda with no calories while fasting. While zero-calorie soda will most likely not affect your fast, it is not the healthiest option overall, so you could take the challenge and minimize it.

Bone broth: It does have a few calories and technically it does break your fast, but many experts are in favor of it, as it contains minerals and electrolytes which you cannot obtain by only having water while you fast. Broth can also be healing for the digestive system if you need to heal your gut. However, research shows that glutamine might prevent your autophagy, so you will need to keep the broth in moderation and not graze on it all day long, but a mug will most likely still be fine.

Healthy fats: There are some people who will take small portions of healthy fats, such as coconut oil or MCT oil while fasting. Technically it does break a fast, but it can curb your cravings and maintain most benefits of intermittent fasting. This is, however, not advised for dieters on weight loss plans, but mostly for those wishing to maintain or slightly change their body composition.

Fruit or fruit juices: It should be going without saying, but for the sake of clarity, fruit or fruit juices will break your fast and load you with carbohydrates, so it's a no while you fast if you want all the benefits of intermittent fasting.

Lemon juice or apple cider vinegar: You can add either to your water to improve the taste, they will not break your fast.

Chewing gum: Many people, myself included, like to chew on gum while fasting. If you want to keep this habit, you will have to opt for a chewing gum without sugar, maybe choose chewing gum with a zero-calorie sweetener. Xylitol, the substance in chewing gum has been found to cause insulin reaction in humans, but unless you plan to chew the whole package of chewing gums in a day, I wouldn't worry about your fast.

So, things aren't that bad, are they? You might find it hard at the beginning to give up your milk and sugar in coffee, but in fact, there are things you can consume to curb a craving and stay strong until it is time for you to break your fast. While this guide is not exhaustive, it can help you understand how the system works and serve you well during your first days of intermittent fasting. When the time to break your fast actually comes, there are ways to do it safely and not impact your body. The right way to break your fast depends on how long you have been fasting for. While a 16-hour fast doesn't need much adaptation when you start eating, a 5-day long fast might need you to take things slower. Many advise in favor of drinking lemon water or water with apple cider vinegar to activate and prepare your digestive system. Bone broth is also a suggested way to break a fast. Bone broth contains collagen and helps you absorb electrolytes better. If you have fasted for over 20 hours it is probably a good idea to drink some bone broth or soup before you have solid food. Some prefer fish broth than bone broth. This is another good alternative, as fish broth contains all the fatty omega 3 acids you need. Your first meal after a fast should be relatively small, about 500 calories. If you are on keto, eggs are always a good idea, as they contain leucine, the amino acid which stimulates muscle growth. If you are not restricting carbs, you can have carbs on your meal but do prefer complex carbs and as unprocessed as you can get. Breaking a fast with fruit is not suggested, as fruit contains a lot of sugars and carbs. If you want to have fruit, you should opt for fruit rich in fiber, such as apples and berries. Meat on the first meal is also not advised. Especially red meat can be hard to digest if you haven't had anything for many hours. You can opt for fish or chicken as your first meal.

However, it is not only fasting which can help activate autophagy as far as diet is concerned. It is considered that a lack of carbohydrates in your system can also stimulate the process. Following a low carb diet, such as keto, seems to further activate your autophagy. This explains why so many people combine the benefits of intermittent fasting and the keto diet. The logic behind it is actually quite simple. As we saw earlier, the body will run on carbohydrates as long as those are available and then switch to fat. While intermittent fasting is one way to take advantage of this principle, the keto diet is an additional helping hand. If we suppose that someone combines intermittent fasting and keto, we have an ideal situation where not only do we have some hours of fasting to activate autophagy, but we also do not have to wait much after our last meal to start burning fat. This happens because the keto diet only has 5% carbs. This means that inevitably the carb deposits will run out very quickly compared to even a dieter who is intermittent fasting but is following a diet with normal or excessive carb intake. The keto diet has been researched into a lot and it also seems to assist people in living with disorders such as epilepsy. Similarly, with fasting, before you begin with the keto diet, always consult your health provider.

A third pillar for the activation of autophagy is exercise. The process of exercising actually causes stressors for your body, as even a too-slight-for-yo-to-notice pressure on a muscle might need attention from your body to heal. Experiments on lab animals have shown that the levels of autophagy after exercise are higher. Exercise is one of the best ways to keep your body cleansed of unnecessary substances. It is not a coincidence that after working out most people feel energetic and euphoric.

So, a small and very brief recap of the three ways to activate autophagy:

1. **Intermittent fasting**
2. **Keto (or low carb)**
3. **Regular exercise**

You can pick one of the three, two of the three or all three together. No matter which diet plan you are following, exercise is important anyway. Keto is very popular at the moment, but many low carb diets have also been popular in recent years. If it is something which works for you, you can combine it with intermittent fasting for even better fat burning results. As far as the exercise is concerned, I know some of you are really not into the exercising thing. Exercise is not the main contributor to your weight loss indeed, this will have to be your diet, but participating in activity can give you better results in that field and also has many other benefits for you, such as activating autophagy.

So, you might ask, if intermittent fasting is not the only way to activate autophagy, why should I bother? Well, IF is not a dietary restriction. It doesn't tell you anything about what you should or shouldn't eat. Will you be able to eat whatever you want? Well, quite frankly, no. Intermittent fasting is not a magic trick, it will not help you lose weight if you don't have a daily caloric deficit. But you can have more satiating meals and less restriction compared to a 6-meals-a-day diet plan, which will give you the chance to overeat 6 times a day, keep you tied to the kitchen meal prepping and make it very easy for you to fall off the wagon at any time your life gets more demanding and doesn't allow you to perform this huge preparation anymore. Actually, let's take a look at some math. If you have an allowance of 1500 calories per day, 6 meals a day means you will have breakfast, lunch, dinner and 3 snacks. If you imagine 1500 calories divided by that many meals, you probably won't have many satiating meals during your nutrition plan. But if there are only 2 meals and 1 snack in your day, like in the 16/8 plan, you immediately have 2 very satiating meals and 1 quite filling snack, and once you get used to the plan, you will rarely feel hungry.

However, as we mentioned earlier, if done improperly or excessively autophagy can be dangerous for the body, so all is to be practiced in moderation. How will you do that you may ask and how will you be sure that you are indeed doing the right thing for your body. Being safe and healthy is always the most important aspect when embarking on a journey which entails changing your lifestyle towards a better body and mind. Find out all about the right and wrong ways to activate autophagy in the next chapter.

Chapter 5: What to Do and Not to Do While Activating Autophagy

Whenever we make changes in our lifestyle, moderation is key. The same holds true when you plan to activate autophagy. While autophagy is indeed a natural procedure which is vital to the survival of our body, excessive autophagy may lead to unpleasant repercussions on your body. Of course, we want to avoid the chance of this happening. Therefore, in this chapter, you will learn all about how to keep autophagy on a beneficial level for your body and not go overboard.

But before we see what you should avoid, one could ask, why excessive autophagy is bad. We already said autophagy is something good, so isn't it common sense that there can't be too much of this good thing? Well, as we said before, the body is a very complex system. While autophagy in moderation is something we really want happening, if we go over the top with it, there might be very negative outcomes. There can be excessive autophagy and this is something we would like to avoid. On the one hand, the process clears the toxic or defective materials of the cells; on the other hand, if the process goes beyond recycling and purifying the proteins, it can begin to destroy the cell, leading to cell death. This means that autophagy should not be excessive. If autophagy clears some proteins that suppress cancer can have negative consequences. This form of excessive autophagy has been named autosis. Autosis is a non-apoptotic form of cell death which depends on the autophagic mechanisms. To put it in simpler words, it is an excessive form of self-digestion which can be dangerous for you. Apoptosis is the scheduled procedure of cell death. It is the natural way in which the body destroys old, dysfunctional or damaged cells and then lets your homeostasis get rid of them with the procedure of phagocytosis. Autosis, on the other hand, does not function in the same way as apoptosis. As the following chart suggests, it can be caused by nutrient depletion, pharmacological reasons or damage, like all the autophagic procedures. However, especially autosis is triggered by starvation, high concentration of autophagy-inducing peptides and neonatal cerebral hypoxia-ischemia.

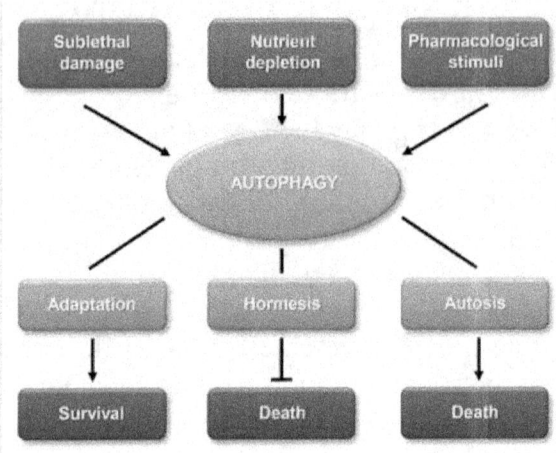

Chart 5.1 - Excessive forms of autophagy

While you activate autophagy, you certainly want to avoid autosis. Therefore, after your fasting periods, you should make sure to load your body with nutrients and energy. Your caloric deficit when you are attempting weight loss should be sustainable. By restricting calories too much, your body might find itself in a position to consider that something really stressful is going on in your environment and end up activating autosis instead of the beneficial autophagy we want to take advantage of. You can calculate your caloric needs and weight loss based on a number of equations, which you can find in the bonus chapter at the end of this book. Another possibility of excessive autophagy is that it might actually have negative results on life expectancy. While the reinforcement of autophagy may be positive for young and middle-aged people, research shows that the function of the mechanism could be negative for the elderly. For example, if autophagy itself starts to malfunction after a certain age, it may be better for it to degrade than to reinforce itself. This idea is based on a study that showed that the cessation of autophagy prolonged the life of the elderly worms by 50%. However, there is no way to be certain about whether this would actually hold true for humans as well and there is not a lot of research evidence proving that autophagy can have a bad effect on the elderly.

Now, about what you should actually do while activating autophagy. We have already discussed the three steps you should follow: fasting, low on carbs and exercise. One way in which autophagy is triggered is to reduce insulin. When we eat, mainly carbohydrates, insulin rises in the blood while glucagon falls. On the other hand, when several hours of a meal pass, insulin falls and glucagon rises. The increase in glucagon (i.e. carbohydrate deficiency) stimulates autophagy and it is no coincidence that this procedure was first described in 1962 when an increase in the number of lysosomes in rat hepatic cells after glucagon injection was observed. Turning on the process requires depletion of nutrients, and modern nutritionists recommend eating no more than three times a day or even skipping our dinner somewhere, as this allows for better detoxification of the cells. The irony is that those who consume juices for detoxification - a fashion of recent years - are undermining the process of autophagy. So, in earlier times, when people were fasting drinking only water, they were right to say they detoxify their bodies. The detox supplements or diets are more often than not worth your time and not beneficial for you. Most of the times all they do is help you lose water weight by visiting the bathroom a tad more often. Especially fruit is rich in carbohydrates, so trying to detox oneself with fruit might give you a big caloric deficit for one or two days, but it will most likely leave you wanting a pizza on the third one and it will not help you activate autophagy.

In addition to fasting, there is another way to boost autophagy which can be used additionally to fasting or by its own: ketosis. It's about taking too few carbohydrates to get the body to use its stored fat. In this way, three molecules are called ketones and used as energy by the brain. Ketosis helps in fat loss and keeps the muscle tissue to a considerable extent. In addition, someone with ketosis can have the benefits of autophagy without having to resort to starvation. The ketogenic diet is high in fat (about 75%) while carbohydrate intake is 5-10% (less than 50 grams per day). Exercise has also been scientifically proven to enhance autophagy. The benefits of aerobic exercise are known for heart and a study published in 2017 found something extra in mice: that it facilitates the removal of dysfunctional mitochondria in heart cells. Indeed, the benefits of exercise disappeared when autophagy was blocked by medication or genetics.

So, what can you do to boost your chances of activating autophagy and avoiding autosis?

Step 1: Determine your caloric needs - You need to keep your body in a stressed state - which you will achieve by fasting, but you also need to actually get through enough energy to maintain a sustainable weight loss rate and not go into excessive autophagy. Nutritionists believe that it is healthy to lose 1% - 1.5% of one's body weight in a week. Therefore, if you weigh 200 lbs., it is safe to lose about 2 lbs. in a week while if you weigh 150 lbs., you would be safe with losing about 1.5 lbs. a week. These numbers may be slightly altered in cases of severely overweight people who need to lose weight imperatively for health reasons. Losing slowly does not always mean that you will not gain back the weight, as it is often suggested. It does, however, hold true to some extent, as a slower and more gradual process is more often than not an indicator of more time to develop healthier habits and overall sustainability.

Step 2: Intermittent fasting - Your model of preference, your preferred hours, everything is your choice. You only need to give your body a minimum of 16 fasting hours every day. It's nothing more than skipping breakfast and having a somewhat late lunch. In the long run, IF will keep you more satiated than a normal eating plan, because, within your 2 or 3 meals/snacks of the day, you can distribute all your caloric allowance and have less but more satiating meals.

Step 3: Lower carb intake - It doesn't have to be keto. Even your normal nutrition plan with some more non-starchy vegetables instead of carbs will be fine. But if you do want to experiment with keto, it is a fact that many combine it with intermittent fasting as the two methods are very compatible. Keto is also a diet which might be restrictive but will more often than not leave you satiated, as it contains medium protein and a lot of fat.

Step 4: Exercise - Exercise goes hand in hand with autophagy. You should remember that exercise apart from many people's favorite pastime and other people's absolute nightmare is nothing more and nothing less than us simulating the activities our species would have to do some thousands of years ago. Running, lifting heavy objects, fighting, and the list could go on and on. Those were stressors which would activate autophagy for people of the era, but for us now, there isn't a chance that we'll need to hunt for our food anytime soon, so we need to create those stressors for ourselves to enhance autophagy.

Chapter 6: Myths and truths about Intermittent Fasting and Autophagy

There are certainly a lot of misconceptions about IF and autophagy. Because I know that you might have been hearing those a lot and even believe some of those, this chapter is dedicated to debunking some of the myths which spread false information about intermittent fasting and autophagy.

Myth #1: Fasting is dangerous

Fasting is in fact not dangerous at all. It has been practiced by people for spiritual, health and other reasons for thousands of years. Pythagoras of Samos, the famous Greek mathematician was said to be an avid fan of fasting. He practiced it for years. St. Catherine was also recorded to have been fasting and the doctors of the Renaissance period were talking of the healing properties of fasting. But history aside, research has also shown that fasting isn't dangerous for you. While there are nutritionists who believe long-term fasting is not a good weight loss tool, because it is not sustainable, intermittent fasting has not received such criticism. It has been found that people who ate over an 8-hour eating window displayed better results than people who followed a normal eating program and they were also not particularly hungry during the process. A study in Alabama showed that perhaps the hours selected for the eating window also matter, but in fact, it is just better that everyone follows the plan which works for them, as long as they can keep in line with their nutrition plan and their activity.

Myth #2: Fasting can lower your blood sugar

Fasting is most likely not to cause any changes in your blood sugar. While it has been observed that in some people blood sugar will rise during a fast, the experts explain that it is only because sugar from the liver flows in your bloodstream. Intermittent fasting is currently being researched as a tool to fight type 2 diabetes. However, some experts believe that fasting is certainly not a tool for diabetics, as the rise in blood sugar after a fast could be too high for them. Here we can see once again that intermittent fasting is not a very groundbreaking form of fasting, it can sustain your normal lifestyle just fine. Fasting for more days is mostly what alarms the experts and is considered to be dangerous for certain groups of people. Bottom line is, if you want to try intermittent fasting, it is most likely you won't face any kind of problems with your blood sugar.

Myth #3: Fasting can cause hormonal imbalances

Fasting itself can only influence your hormones to a certain extent. This is why if you know you have hormonal issues, such as thyroid problems, you should always reach out to your health provider before you start on this regime. As far as the hormones of hunger and fat-storing are concerned, IF seems to have very good results at stimulating ghrelin, which improves brain dopamine levels and to put it simply, makes you feel better. Another more heated area of discussion is estrogen and progesterone, the hormones which are important for the menstrual cycle in females. While women can follow intermittent fasting, they might be more sensitive than men because they have more kisspeptin. If done incorrectly, intermittent fasting can cause problems in the menstrual cycle. This is why for women, it is suggested that they do not fast for 2 consecutive days in a week and if they are on intermittent fasting on a daily basis, they work with a 12-16 hour fast. What might also be useful is to start with a 12/12 model - which doesn't offer much in terms of results, but helps get you in the mentality of IF - , go on with a 14/10 and then reach the 16/8 to have a more gradual adaptive process.

Myth #4: Fasting can lead to stress

Many people trying to decide on whether they will try intermittent fasting or not are worried it may cause them excessive stress. Fasting is a stressor on the body, but so is exercise. In the right doses, fasting won't cause any excess stress. However, what is true to some extent is that IF may not be for people who have an adrenal imbalance or are struggling with their circadian rhythm. Your circadian rhythm is the periodic way in which you do things in your day. For instance, if you always sleep at 10 pm and wake up at 7 am, it is highly likely that by now your body has adjusted to it and feels sleepy at 10 pm. People who face trouble with this have been observed to have trouble handling an intermittent fasting regime. However, this is due to the fact that the individual has stress problems before going on that eating plan, the intermittent fasting itself is not to blame for excess stress. If you are a person suffering from excess stress, that does not mean that you should rule out intermittent fasting before giving it a shot. An easy regime such as the 16/8 could be a great fit for you. Furthermore, you can take other steps such as meditation, yoga, spirituality to alleviate stress and further contribute to your weight loss.

Myth #5: Fasting can cause overeating

Many people fear that if they start intermittent fasting, they're going to overeat because they will feel the need to overcompensate for the meal(s) they have skipped. Overcompensating for skipping a meal is actually a myth, as research has shown. It is very sensible to suggest that you will eat more for the meals you are allowed to have, but this would rarely add up to being equal in energy as the meal you have skipped or throwing you off your caloric allowance. If you do find yourself overeating or binging during your intermittent fasting journey, take a step back and see whether you have tried to fast for too many hours without preparation and whether your energy intake from the previous days was enough to keep you going. It is not uncommon for people embarking on a weight loss journey to be very strict with themselves at first and then loosen up in the next days, but if you are intermittent fasting, you will need to eat mindfully to avoid eating too little or too much.

Myth #6: Fasting can burn muscle mass

Actually, research has proved the following. Two recent studies conducted in 2010 and 2016 showed that intermittent fasting didn't cause muscle loss to the participants in the one, while in the other the control group which was only restricting calories lost more muscle mass over the course of the research than the IF group. Intermittent fasting doesn't burn muscle mass. In fact, it seems to preserve lean tissue more than other diet methods.

Myth #7: You can't work out while fasting

This is a very popular myth. There is some grain of truth in the fact that you can't engage in too strenuous physical activity while fasting, but your everyday workout will not be a problem. On the contrary, many fitness professionals and amateurs swear by working out while fasting. This actually has a name, working out in a fasted state, and it is considered to be making your workout even more effective and assisting your fat loss. Some suggest that you should only have caffeine and green tea before said workout for the best results. Many IF dieters prefer to break their fast after their workout. What is most important is to listen to one's own body. Maybe your first days of intermittent fasting will be hard to follow and you may find yourself not feeling energetic enough to exercise, but in the long run, you can find both the IF model and the ideal exercise for you. If this is your first time attempting weight loss, the first few days might be challenging and leave you sleepy, lacking energy. But it is only what happens at first, it will improve by itself during the next couple of days. Just be patient and think of your goal. It is a better lifestyle you are opening your body and mind to.

Myth #8: Fasting equals weight loss

This is a very common misconception which can be attributed to some marketing strategies used by various stakeholders to sell products related to intermittent fasting. Especially at the beginning of this new emergence of fasting as a weight management method, there were many who shamelessly promoted intermittent fasting as a way to lose weight without counting calories. While it is true that an 8-hour eating window gives you fewer chances of going over the top and therefore you may feel more confident and free about your meals of choice, grazing on low quality caloric dense processed foods for 8 hours will make you gain weight despite the best of your efforts to keep up with your eating window. Calories in - calories out hasn't been debunked to this day, contrary to what many people who want to sell you something want you to believe. It is pure physics, there are about 3500 calories in a pound of fat, therefore to lose a pound you need to accumulate a caloric deficit of 3500 calories over a certain amount of days. While fasting is a very nice and helpful way to monitor your eating, the food choices are still of paramount importance. As we were taught in high school, there is no energy which can be created from thin air, nor can energy disappear into thin air. You will need to create and maintain your deficit throughout the entire weight loss period. Fasting is a tool which can help you and will certainly have more benefits for your body than conventional weight loss, but it is no magic pill. Weight loss will require a significant amount of planning and effort on your behalf - but do not let this dishearten you! The work you have to do for it is what will make you proud in the end and remind you that you should not neglect your nutrition, even if you reach your body goals.

Myth #9: Fasting will send you into starvation mode

This is probably the point where we get back to the old starvation mode myth. The premise is simple, if you're not eating at least every 4-6 hours, your body will go into starvation mode and you won't be able to lose weight anymore. There is no evidence to suggest that happens at all. While we do know that adaptive thermogenesis exists and the body will, in fact, do some things to avoid losing weight, the numbers are not enough to suggest that this is the reason you are not losing weight or even gaining it. The Minnesota starvation experiment, which is always credited as a source of why starvation mode is real, in fact, didn't prove anything like that. The participants by the end of the program had lost 25% of their body weight and hit 5% body fat by following a regime of two meals per day and more caloric restriction than most of the diets we do. The experiment resulted in saying that starvation mode is true because the participants had a 40% average reduction in metabolism. However, only a small part of this was adaptive. Most of the change was due to the fact that these people had lost a lot of weight, so naturally, their body didn't burn that much energy to keep them functioning anymore. And if the starvation mode was by any chance true, why do we have all these overwhelming and very sad pictures from wartime or disease which show emaciated people? If there was truth to the starvation mode, these people shouldn't have been able to lose any more weight when the food became too little - but unfortunately, they did, and many of them died of starvation. Fasting will not send you into starvation mode. It is very probable that if you have at some point in your life stopped losing weight and found no better explanation than the starvation mode, the truth is you were either underestimating your food intake or overestimating the calories your burned during exercise. It has happened to the best of us. If you have trouble with your weight loss, do not blame it on starvation mode. Keep a food and exercise diary for a week and then check if the math adds up. If it does not, you might need to check with your health provider, but most of the times it will add up.

Chapter 7: Benefits of Intermittent Fasting and Autophagy

Almost everyone does intermittent fasting at least in part for fat loss and that's one of the biggest benefits of intermittent fasting. It keeps your insulin level low for more total hours a day and that helps you lose fat, as it helps your body remember "I can also burn fat!". Intermittent fasting helps your body remember that your brain can also burn fat for fuel it does not have to just burn glucose like at many of us were taught in health as well. So, as you begin intermittent fasting you are going to burn fat and that's good if you're trying to lose weight. When the stomach is empty, the body quickly changes hormone levels to gain access to stored body fat. It sheds insulin levels in the blood to ease fat burning and increases growth hormones in the blood to a much higher level to burn fat and develop muscles, thereby accelerating the cellular process and bringing about changes in the various genes and molecules related to immunity and longevity.

Intermittent fasting is also used with amazing success to treat type 2 diabetes. One of the main causes of type 2 diabetes is insulin resistance. High blood sugar levels can be adjusted by removing or reducing insulin resistance. Many of the studies have shown one of the biggest benefits of intermittent fasting is the ability to lower the sugar

level by 3% -6% and insulin resistance by 20% -
31%. Type 2 diabetics when they start to
implement intermittent fasting will have
immediate and noticeable weight loss as well as an
immediate improvement in their hemoglobin A1c
and their other lab values. People who have lost a
ton of weight on a high carb starvation diet might
get angry or hungry and even if they manage to
lose the weight can have a lot of loose skin or
redundant skin. Intermittent fasting may help you
lose weight and avoid the excess skin -- of course,
that depends on the amount of weight too --
because of a process called autophagy.

But intermittent fasting is not only for people who
want to lose weight. People who go to the gym
often claim that they can tell it helps them with
their gain. There is research that shows that
intermittent fasting increases your human growth
hormone - which is pretty much the hormone of
the gym - to help you gain muscle and be as
effective as possible. But even when someone is
not going to the gym but performs manual labor
instead, they might notice that they are getting
stronger and their daily activities become easier.
Therefore, muscle growth and elevated HGH levels
are definitely a byproduct of intermittent fasting.

Another benefit of intermittent fasting is improved
immunity. Many people who have adopted this
lifestyle observe that they no longer get sick as
much. Because of the intermittent fasting your
immune system and your immune response is in
better shape and so you're just better able to either

not get sick or if you do get sick it's a much milder illness and it goes away quicker. You have to keep in mind the human body has a very good adjusting capability. When the body is being fed constantly or very often, the immune system may be underworking. The body knows that there is a lot of energy going around so it is less likely to be productive and keep you in top shape and energy, knowing that soon it will be fed again, so no additional effort is required. On the other hand, when you are fasting there are quite a few hours - depending on your intermittent fasting protocol- when your body feels you are not getting enough food. "We are hungry", your body thinks. No, this is not starvation mode. It is the fasting mode. Thinking that it is hungry and that the next meal might be far away - because humans were initially supposed to hunt and collect food, not open the fridge or order takeout - the body does its very best to keep you energetic and assist you in being productive and making sure that you are doing well. Your immune system is working well and it's ready to tackle any problems before they actually become a full-blown illness. Some of the scientific findings show that heart health can be improved through a regular fasting program as it addresses many risk factors such as inflammation markers, sugar levels, triglycerides, LDL cholesterol level, etc. There are also many positive animal research results to reduce the risk of developing cancer as well as limiting the side effects of chemotherapy.

Moreover, fasting has always been associated with longevity. News from the research field is very encouraging, as every animal that scientists have ever fasted in the lab lives up to 30 to 50% longer. A new study from Harvard has found that intermittent fasting can prolong life, as it slows down the aging of the cells by altering the way mitochondrial networks function inside the cell. So, there is a very good chance that if you want to live a longer, fuller life intermittent fasting is the answer to your question.

Intermittent fasting is always being associated with higher levels of energy and concentration. Many people also feel physically stronger while fasting and they prefer to have their workouts before they break their fast. Intermittent fasting has also been linked with a decrease in inflammation. Research on 50 healthy adults has shown that the participants who opted for intermittent fasting for one month had a decrease in inflammatory markers.

Intermittent Fasting or Caloric Restrictive Diet?

This debate seems to always be present when it comes to intermittent fasting. While research has shown that as far as weight loss is concerned, both methods can have similar results, we could not forget the other added benefits intermittent fasting has for our health. Many argue that IF is not a sustainable plan, but I beg to differ. A huge amount of people has been skipping breakfast and having a late lunch and it seems that if it suits one's lifestyle, it is not unsustainable at all in the long run. While intermittent fasting does not mean you can eat whatever you feel like, it promotes a mindful eating mindset. While on a restrictive diet you could spend a significant amount of your day counting calories, intermittent fasting gives you a relative sense of freedom, but you still need to make good choices.

Last but not least, as previously said, intermittent fasting stimulates autophagy. While a low carb diet might be hard to follow for most, intermittent fasting doesn't take much adaptation and can be followed by anyone. On a practical level, it saves much time otherwise required for meal planning and it helps you have more satiating meals and not obsess over calorie counting while you make your nutrition plans. Intermittent fasting has all the health benefits we discussed earlier, so it is indeed a smart choice over a traditional diet and it can accommodate your lifestyle and the social events you will want to attend in your nutrition plan much easier.

Benefits of Autophagy

Stimulating autophagy will offer you many things: it clears out recent, unwanted cellular materials and proteins, and it conjointly stimulates the assembly of human growth hormone, that regenerates contemporary cellular material and fuels up cell renewal. If your body has recently had an infection, autophagy is also ready to destroy lingering microorganism or viruses. Autophagy isn't solely joined to increasing longevity, it's serving to researchers to raised understanding chronic diseases like Parkinson's and Alzheimer's. In case autophagy doesn't happen often, the body collects a spread of cellular material, together with proteins that show up in giant quantities in Alzheimer's, Parkinson's, and even cancer. Researchers believe that prolonged bouts of autophagy can be ready to clear the brain of these excess proteins, therefore probably preventing the event of these diseases.

Life could not have existed for a long time without the process of autophagy. When cell sensors detect low availability of nutrients, they "tell" cells to stop growing and begin to break down unnecessary parts: this is essentially the path of self-purification, of autophagy. When the process does not work properly, harmful proteins can accumulate.

The question is whether boosting fasting through fasting or a fasting diet like a ketogenic diet can prevent or help with treating certain diseases. An area of interest is neurodegenerative diseases e.g. Alzheimer, Parkinson, and Huntington. These diseases are characterized by excessive accumulation of proteins within the neurons leading to dysfunction - the neurons are non-replaceable cells. The failure of protein degradation pathways can play an important role in the prevention of these diseases; however, its exact role has not yet been clarified. Other studies indicate that some diseases may be due to mitochondrial dysfunction, such as e.g. heart failure. Mitochondria are -- as we so often heard in school biology -- "the powerhouse of the cell". This explains why their function is so important for your health, as any system is unable to run properly without being fueled well. So, in these cases, autophagy can play an important role. Note that a study showed that even depression is associated with a dysfunction of the mitochondria.

With regard to diabetes, a study done in mice showed that a diet that imitates fasting - and featuring periods of feeding and hunger - can reverse diabetes and actually regenerate the pancreas. The cause of this is not known but could be related to autophagy. The lead of the experiment was Valter Longo, a professor of gerontology, and what the researchers found was that with hunger and feeding cycles, beta cells were produced in the pancreas that produced insulin. Beta cells detect glucose in the blood and release insulin when sugar levels are high. With the restoration of pancreatic function, diabetic symptoms were reversed.

Some researchers consider autophagy as a factor which reduces the risk of cancer. While there is no scientific evidence to support this, some studies suggest that indeed the risk for cancer could be reduced through autophagy. In 2018, Dr Kyriakopoulos conducted a research on the matter and reached the conclusion that based on autophagy's property to All existing surveys in the field of autophagy indicate that it can affect the resolution process as far as alterations in DNA are concerned and that it plays an important role in relation to damage and DNA repair. One of the most interesting things is that it remains unclear is whether autophagy is helping to repair damaged DNA or it suspends its repair to keep the entire body safe. In general lines, if the damage can be corrected, the autophagy mechanism promotes its restoration. Alternatively, when there is irreparable damage, autophagy can lead to the initiation of cell death programs, including apoptosis and autophagy-related cell death. Further studies are needed to reveal this exciting but still vague role of autophagy in the repair process of DNA. However, it does seem that there is evidence to suggest that autophagy plays a key role in the cytotoxic function of your immune system - this is exactly the process which destroys damaged cells, and in other words, your built-in defense against cancer and DNA damage.

Autophagy is a homeostatic mechanism for quality control of the life and the fate of the cell. When it comes to tumorigenesis, it is not clear whether autophagy helps reduce the risk of cancer, but there is a distinct possibility that this is true. At the moment, there are indications that both autophagy as well as DNA repair are associated with the effectiveness of chemotherapy or radiotherapy and have an important role in non-response in cancer therapies. In the future, it will be of paramount importance to further investigate the interaction between autophagy and DNA repair in order to achieve greater efficacy in the treatment of cancer.

I certainly hope this chapter has enlightened you on all the health benefits this journey has to offer to you. Apart from the weight loss and fat loss, the significantly less loose skin compared to people who follow a conventional diet, you will also find yourself struggling much less with inflammation, while your immune system will be functioning better than ever. Activating the process of autophagy brings about another set of very important benefits. Autophagy can help you in your fight against diabetes, reduce your risk of cancer and other diseases and keep your body in top shape against any threat from the outside. There is no reason why you wouldn't like to swap or combine any existing weight loss plan you have with intermittent fasting. But you might say, all this sounds very good in theory. But is intermittent fasting the right plan for me? This is what we'll talk about on the next chapter, where you'll also find a test on which intermittent fasting protocol would be the best for you regarding your own lifestyle and choices.

Chapter 8: Is it for Me?

Intermittent fasting, as it can be seen by the benefits chapter, can be very good for your health and nutrition. But that doesn't mean you can make it work for your lifestyle. Therefore, I have gathered some of the positive and negative comments people have been making about intermittent fasting. After all, science is accurate but if you want a sustainable method to manage your weight and change your lifestyle, it should definitely be a model which can work for you. Just like in all other fields, in weight loss there isn't a one size fits all, and there isn't one in intermittent fasting as well.

After all this analysis you might be wondering, is intermittent fasting for you? The health benefits are many and desirable, but is this the method which will guide you to the better you? I have created this short test for you to find out which IF models could work best for you and your own lifestyle. Take the results of the test with a grain of salt, as this book isn't meant to substitute medical advice. Though intermittent fasting and autophagy are procedures you can follow without a great amount of monitoring, make sure to check with your nutritionist or general doctor before you decide to alter your eating style by adopting intermittent fasting.

But before we move on to the test, let's see some pros and cons of intermittent fasting according to people who have tried it or health experts. Most people who have tried intermittent fasting regimes are very pleased with the sense of freedom they have about their nutrition. Being freed from having to meal prep for 6 meals a day and obsessing over not going over your caloric allowance when you have to eat said 6 meals seems to be a very good element of intermittent fasting for most dieters. While a caloric deficit is the only way to lose weight, it seems that intermittent fasting, once you get the hang of it, makes it look more effortless. The only thing you have to do is not break your fast and not make extremely unhealthy choices during your eating window. Compare that to restricting and counting calories 24/7. It's very rational that dieters nowadays have drifted far away from the 6 meals a day model and opt for alternatives like IF.

The general feeling of wellbeing which is experienced by people on IF is also one of the most convincing positive elements. People tend to feel energetic while fasting, their immune system is working perfectly. They observe that winter is going by and they haven't gotten sick at all like they used to. Fasting does stimulate your immune system and gives your body just the right amount of stress to be ready for any possible threat from the environment.

One of the best properties of fasting is that it helps you reconnect with your real sense of hunger. Many people who face problems with weight management have forgotten how to listen to their body. They sometimes find themselves unable to identify whether they are actually hungry or simply craving something or wishing to eat out of boredom. With intermittent fasting, you will have some long fasting periods which will make you feel hungry again and experience how that really feels - like we so rarely have the chance to experience nowadays. While this may be scaring you, hunger in intermittent fasting context does not equal deprivation, as soon enough you will be able to break your fast and have a bigger meal than you could have on a traditional diet plan. Most people who have been on intermittent fasting for a long time no longer face trouble with not breaking their fast. And if one day you break it, this too is okay. Who would claim to never have cheated on a traditional diet? You can always start over on the next day with a better knowledge of what makes you have cravings and when in the day you usually feel hungry.

So, you might ask, are there no shortcomings to intermittent fasting? While it is true that intermittent fasting is a very well thought out lifestyle with many ways to follow it, especially beginners might have trouble on the first days. You might feel sleepy or underfed, but this is only normal while your body adjusts to the new eating schedule. It shouldn't last more than 3 - 5 days. There is certain research which points out intermittent fasting isn't necessarily better than a normal diet for weight loss, but it has many added health benefits and it is way more convenient than your normal 6 meals a day diet.

While IF is a very beneficial method of weight management, it is certainly not for everyone. It has been proven that due to biochemical reasons, men fast better than women. That doesn't mean women should not intermittent fast, they should just be more careful with giving their body the time to adjust and not going too harsh on themselves. While there is much discussion about whether diabetics should fast, there isn't scientific evidence to suggest the opposite. There has been quite some research on pregnant women and whether they should fast, but it remains inconclusive, with most nutritionists being in favor of eating whenever the mother is hungry to ensure proper fetal development. There is no direct evidence to suggest that intermittent fasting could harm the fetus, but there have been observations of premature births in women who followed the Ramadan fast, which consists of dry fasting for 12-20 hours a day, from sunrise to sunset. Fasting is not recommended for anyone under the age of 18, but recently some new articles are reconsidering, saying that probably teenagers wouldn't face any problems caused by intermittent fasting. However, minors who think they should be going on this plan had better check with their physician. Intermittent fasting is not for anyone with an eating disorder, as it could be your way to further restricting yourself and worsening your health condition. If you are an individual with an eating disorder reading this book, you are kindly advised to seek out help for the disordered behavior before researching any diets, eating regimes or nutrition plans.

Now, you have already been given a lot of information to take in, but I'm sure what you're most thinking about is the IF plans and which one is the ideal plan for you. This is why I designed this small test to help you find out which plan you can accommodate better in your lifestyle and would probably be a good match for you. Of course, this test is not medical advice and it should not be regarded as such. It is only a suggestion based on your lifestyle. It won't take you long at all, it is only 10 questions long. Take down your answers on a virtual or real notepad, because you will need them to calculate your score by the end of the test and of course, be honest!

Test - Which IF plan should you choose?

Question 1: Have you tried intermittent fasting before?

a) Yes, and I had no trouble adjusting.

b) Yes, but it was not easy.

c) No.

Question 2: How would you describe your time for meal planning?

a) A lot.
b) Barely enough.
c) Not enough.

Question 3: Do you feel hungry often?

a) Very often.
b) Sometimes.
c) Not really.

Question 4: How would you describe your lifestyle?

a) Sedentary
b) Quite busy
c) Very busy

Question 5: How many meals (count snacks too) do you usually get through in a day?

a) 2 or 3

b) 3 or 4

c) More than 4

Question 6: Have you been on a weight loss regime before?

a) Yes, and still on it.

b) Yes, and now maintaining.

c) No.

Question 7: How would you describe your relationship with overeating?

a) I never overeat.

b) I sometimes overeat.

c) I often overeat.

Question 8: Have you found yourself binging on food?

a) Many times.

b) Only once or twice.

c) Never.

Question 9: How would you describe your relationship with food and nutrition?

a) Healthy.
b) Could be better.
c) Unhealthy.

Question 10: Do you have any hormonal issues or a menstrual cycle?

Question	1 point	2 points	3 points
1	c	b	a
2	a	b	c
3	a	b	c
4	a	b	c
5	c	b	a
6	a	b	c
7	c	b	a
8	a	b	c

9	c	b	a
10	c	b	a

a) Never had any issues and I don't have a menstrual cycle.

b) I have a menstrual cycle but no hormonal issues.

c) I have sometimes faced hormonal imbalances.

Calculate your score based on this table:

So, as you probably notice after calculating your score, the minimum you might have scored is 10 points and the maximum 30 points. Based on that:

10 - 16 points: You are probably a beginner in the world of intermittent fasting or someone who has been struggling with weight loss and their relationship with food on many levels before deciding to take up intermittent fasting. Perhaps the best plan for you would be one which will give you the necessary time to adapt and see if this method works for you and how you can make it sustainable. This is why my suggestion for you would be to start on the 16/8 plan. It will keep you eating quite frequently compared to other IF regimes and if you see it works for you and you can curb your hunger, you can work your way up to more demanding protocols.

17 - 23 points: You have had quite a few weight loss or nutrition plan experiences in your life and maybe even experimented with intermittent fasting before. If you are a beginner with IF, you can try the 16/8 plan as a base. However, if you are more experienced, if you have no problem regulating your eating window and your lifestyle doesn't leave you much time for meal prepping, maybe the best plan for you would be 5:2 (or its variation, "Eat - Stop - Eat"). This plan will save you from having to meal prep for about 2 days of the week and still let you enjoy normal quantities of food in your 5 feeding days. If the 24-hour fast seems scary, start with the 5:2 which contains some few calories even on the 2 fasting days.

24 - 30 points: You are probably in a position where you have already tried a lot of things with your body and you know by now how to make them work for you. Because you do have a way of controlling what goes into your body and a healthy relationship with food, any IF plan would most likely cause you no problem. If you also happen to be a quite busy individual, maybe it's time to try OMAD or the Warrior Diet. A very small eating window which will only have you meal planning for one very generous meal every day will probably not be a problem for you. If, however, a fast longer than 20 hours every day seems like something you wouldn't like to do, you are always welcome to try "Eat - Stop - Eat".

Chapter 9: Tips and Recipes

If you already made it this far in the book, it means you have quite a lot of determination to start on your new lifestyle and discover what is best for your body. It also means you were able to read various information based on science, history and many other fields and you have assumed by now a very good base knowledge about intermittent fasting and how you can use it to activate your autophagy. But even with all your determination, every start can be hard and changing your eating habits may certainly give you some trouble. Therefore, for the few brave ones who made it this far, I have gathered plenty of useful tips for your own intermittent fasting plan. And not only that but also a few recipes which you can use to have a healthy dinner when you break your fast. Among those, you will find low-carb recipes and also vegetarian and vegan recipes for the ones with dietary restrictions.

Tips

Tip #1: Use your schedule wisely.

Most of us take 7-8 hours of sleep at night. Those are about 8 hours of fasting during which you won't feel hungry at all, because you will be sleeping. If you want to start with, let's say, the 16/8 plan, using your sleeping time wisely is key. If you can bring yourself not to snack after dinner on the previous night and skip breakfast, you have 16 hours of fasting which have gone by relatively easily. A late lunch and a somewhat late dinner with one snack in between will not leave you hungry. This does not only hold true for the 16/8 model. It all depends on your own lifestyle. If you know that one day of your week is going to be so busy that you will barely have time to breathe, you can have your 24-hour fast on that day by stopping your eating after last night's dinner and resuming it to give yourself a nice satiating dinner on the day in question. If you have a very active daytime job, you may find yourself trying OMAD or the Warrior Diet.

Tip #2: Eat mindfully.
Intermittent fasting is a wonderful and powerful tool, but it is only a tool. You can use it to facilitate your progress and improve your performance, but if you want to lose weight, you will have to combine it with your nutrition plan. If you are unsure of what to eat to lose weight in a healthy and sustainable way, do not hesitate to see a nutritionist who will come up with suggestions based on your preferences and your nutritional needs. Eating mindfully doesn't have to be a process of weighing your portions and counting calories, as more experienced dieters will often have no problem eyeballing their portions and they will know which foods to avoid and which to go for. But if you are new to the world of nutrition, a food scale could be a very good investment which will give you doubt free cooking and serving sizes for a lifetime.

Tip #3: Work out in a fasted state
As mentioned before, many people swear by it and it can apparently boost your fat loss and the effectiveness of your workout. Many find that during their fasting period they feel more energetic and concentrated as well and therefore they plan their workouts accordingly.

Tip #4: Be patient.
"The start is a good half of everything," said the ancient Greeks, and they were very right. Deciding to start on a new lifestyle is very important. But you have to remember, every start is difficult. You might feel hungry or tired and lose heart, but remember, it will only get easier as time goes by and soon it will feel like second nature.

Tip #5: Find your support system.
It is always a good idea to enlist more helpers in your weight loss journey, especially if you are not experienced with nutrition. Losing weight with a good friend or a family member can keep both of you more motivated. However, even experienced people will find that keeping up with their healthy lifestyle becomes easier and more pleasant when they share it. Find a fitness pal, enroll in cooking classes with a friend or your significant other. It will help you keep up with your nutrition plan even when you feel demotivated.

Tip #6: Find the best model for you.
The best IF model for you doesn't have to be the model that works for your best friend. It doesn't

have to be the model that works for your favorite YouTuber. You should feel free to experiment and find what works best for you and your own lifestyle. It's okay to make mistakes and you can always start over until you find the best plan for you.

Tip #7: When hungry, blunt your appetite.
When starting on a fasting regime, sometimes you will inevitably feel hunger. What you can do to power through this feeling and not break your fast is rely on zero-calorie liquids, which will fill you up and help you buy some time until it's time for your next meal. When unsure of which drinks will not break your fast, check out chapter 4, where you will find specific information about most liquids people tend to ask about.

Tip #8: Keep yourself busy.
This might seem like a strange piece of advice concerning weight loss, but research has shown that boredom is a factor why many people tend to overeat. The reason behind that is dopamine. Dopamine is responsible for reward-motivated behavior and makes you feel good. Boredom leaves us wanting to feel good, therefore eating is a very familiar response. We tend to overeat on snacks and load on useless calories when we feel bored. This is mindless eating; we don't even enjoy it so much but we just do it out of boredom. A full bag of chips while you're watching Netflix, a highly-processed snack while you wait for your flight to board or the dreaded doughnut box when you're tired and bored at work may challenge your weight

loss in the long run. Therefore, especially when you recognize that you are only looking for something to eat because of boredom, you should give yourself things to do. Many people find that starting a hobby helps their weight loss attempts by giving them another outlet to feel good rather than food.

Tip #9: Keep enjoying life.
Intermittent fasting is not only popular because of its positive effects on health, but also because it can fit into our lifestyle very well, unlike other eating plans. Many people will refuse to go to social occasions when on a diet, afraid of cheating on their plan. With intermittent fasting, you will still need to eat healthily, but you can work your way into incorporating some unhealthy foods into your diet on special occasions. Is it your best friend's birthday party? You can skip breakfast and have a light lunch, and here you have it. You can taste the food and even have some cake, and if you're being mindful, you can still be in a caloric deficit at the end of the day. Going on vacation? You can add some more walking to your plan and by skipping breakfast you can have a good taste of the local cuisine in two meals later in the day. Such small treats will help you avoid the black and white mentality. You have probably fallen for this trap many times while dieting. Loading on unhealthy foods before day 1 of your nutrition plan or making a poor food choice and then letting the entire day escape from your control, feeling that you have already ruined it, are actions which do not help you. On the contrary, they take away your

enjoyment of life and they make your relationship with food even worse. Moderation is the key to keep enjoying yourself, sticking to your diet plan without feeling deprived and holding on to your sanity!

Tip #10 - There are no forbidden foods.

But carbs? But fats? But, am I allowed to eat pizza on a diet? May I have cake? Well, in fact, no food is so powerful that a single serving in the right frequency can mess up your entire nutrition plan. You can afford to eat anything, provided that you can fit it in your nutrition plan. Are you craving a burger with fries? Well, let's be frank, it's definitely not your healthiest choice and you can't be having one each day if you're serious about your fat loss. But planning to have a burger with fries on a Saturday evening by cutting 200 calories from your allowance every day of the week leading to that will still keep you in the same caloric deficit overall. However, you should establish your limits to how often you will bend your rules. Don't fall for the infamous cheat day, as one full day of eating processed and caloric dense foods can threaten your weekly caloric deficit. Instead of that, you can opt for one cheat meal per week and make sure to accommodate it in your allowance. This will keep you away from the forbidden food mentality, show you in practice that moderation is key and ultimately help you achieve your goals and be sustainable.

Recipes

No matter how experienced or inexperienced you are with cooking, a nutrition plan will more often than not leave you wanting some new recipes, bored with eating the same things every day. Therefore, in this last part of the book, you will find a few recipes which can combine your weight loss goals with your brand new intermittent fasting schedule. Feel free to experiment, change things around and remember, cooking is supposed to be fun!

Eggplant boats with onion, tomato and feta cheese (Low carb, Vegetarian/Vegan).

Makes 6-8 servings
About 295 calories per serving
Preparation time: 30'
Cooking time: 65'

While it does take some time to make, this Mediterranean inspired dish can also be served cold, so it could be an MVP in your meal planning!

Ingredients:
8 eggplants
4 medium-sized onions
Parsley
Thyme
Cumin
Garlic, crushed, 1 clover

400 gr. Tomato Concasse
Salt and pepper
400 gr. Feta cheese (If cooking vegan, you can omit
this or replace it with a substitute)
Olive oil

How To:
1. Preheat the oven to 350 F.
2. With a knife, we make three horizontal cuts on each eggplant on one side.
3. We open them a little with our hands, careful not to break them, and add salt and pepper.
4. Put the eggplants on a baking tray and bake for 40 minutes.
5. Place a pan on medium to high fire.
6. Cut the onions into thin slices.
7. Once the pan is hot, add 4 tablespoons of olive oil and the onions.
8. When the onions are sautéed, add the garlic.
9. Add cumin, salt, pepper and sauté over low heat for 15-20 minutes until the onions are caramelized.
10. Add the tomato concasse and thyme and mix. Remove from the fire.
11. Serve with parsley and chunks of feta cheese on top. Enjoy!

Zucchini gazpacho (Low carb, Vegan)

Makes 6-8 servings
About 57 calories in each serving
Preparation time: 20'
Cooking time: 20'

A super quick and tasty recipe. You can consume it to break your fast and give your digestive system a heads up before you attempt a bigger or heavier meal.

Ingredients:
3 tbsp. olive oil
3 leeks, the white piece
1 pc. garlic
4 zucchini, cut into 2 cm pieces
Juice of 2 lemons
700 g water
10 basil leaves + extra for serving
Salt and pepper
¼ tbsp chili flakes for serving.

How To:
1. Heat the olive oil in a pan on medium heat.
2. Cut the white piece of leeks into thin slices and sauté for 5-6 minutes until they soften but they do not get very brown.
3. Remove the pan from the fire, transfer the leeks to a bowl, and allow to cool for 20 minutes.
4. Transfer the leek to a blender along with garlic, zucchini, lemon juice, water, basil leaves, salt, and pepper.
5. Beat for 1-2 minutes until we have a uniform and smooth blend.
6. Serve with chili flakes and basil leaves.

Salad with lentils and beetroots (Vegan)

Makes 6-8 servings
About 226 calories in a serving
Preparation time: 20'
Cooking time: 20'

This hearty salad contains lentils, a very good source of protein. Whether you follow the vegan lifestyle or not, such a recipe is very good to break your fast and could also serve as a nice and healthy side for your next dinner party!

Ingredients:
3 liters of water
1 bay leaf
200 g tricolor lentils
400 g celery
Juice from one lemon
2 beets (boiled)
40 g hazelnuts
Parsley

For the dressing:
20 g vinegar
1 tbsp. mustard
1 tbsp. honey or agave syrup
Salt and pepper
20 g olive oil
50 g sunflower oil
parsley, chopped, for serving

How To:

1. In a saucepan, add 1.5 liters of water, bay leaf, and lentils and boil for 10-15 minutes.
2. Drain the lentils and put them in a large bowl.
3. Cut the celery root into 2-3 cm cubes.
4. Boil the remaining water (1.5 liters) in a pot.
5. Pour the juice from the lemon and boil the celery root for 15-20 minutes until it softens. Strive it and put it in the bowl.
6. Clean and cut the beets in irregular slices, cut the hazelnuts in the middle and put them in the bowl.
7. Chop the parsley and put it in the bowl.

For the dressing:
1. In a bowl, add the vinegar, mustard, honey, salt, and pepper.
2. Beat well with a hand mixer to homogenize and gradually pour the olive oil first and then the sunflower oil.
3. Add the dressing to the bowl of vegetables, mix with a wooden spoon and serve with chopped parsley.

Chicken spinach salad with pomegranate

Makes 6-8 servings
About 390 calories per serving
Preparation time: 20'
Cooking time: 10'

A chicken salad is a nice way to break your fast, but this one is a whole meal by itself. If you're going low carb, you can omit or replace the fruit. Featuring a healthy and delicious dressing which will surely be your favorite soon!

Ingredients:
2 cups baby spinach leaves
2 chicken breasts
½ cup arugula (optional for the fans of the taste)
Seeds from one pomegranate
1/2 cup Walnuts
Grape tomatoes (optional, for serving)
An orange
Parmesan cheese
Sweet paprika
Salt and pepper

For the dressing:
¼ cup mayonnaise
¼ cup Greek yogurt
1 tbsp honey

How To:
1. Preheat the oven at 400F.

2. Cut the chicken in cubes or strips. Salt and pepper generously. Add sweet paprika.
3. On a baking tray, line the chicken, put in the oven and let cook until golden brown.
4. Finely chop the orange in small cubes.
5. Toss the spinach, arugula, orange, pomegranate seeds, and walnuts.
6. Add the chicken when cooked. Top with parmesan cheese shavings.
7. For the dressing, combine the mayonnaise, Greek yogurt, and honey.
8. Serve with grape tomatoes.

Stuffed tomatoes with rice (Vegan)

Makes 4-6 servings
About 255 calories in a serving
Preparation time: 40'
Cooking time: 100'

Though there are variations of this recipe containing ground beef or shrimp, the only rice version is more trouble-free and fit for your vegan friends! You can serve with cheese or cheese substitute for some more protein. This very practical dish can be eaten both warm and cold, do keep it in mind for your meal preps!

Ingredients:
10 medium-sized tomatoes
1 cup of rice
2 big onions
2 garlic cloves
1 tsp sugar
Olive oil
Parsley
Spearmint
Salt and pepper
2 big potatoes (optional)

How To:
1. Cut a slice on the top and remove the insides from the tomatoes. Make sure not to break them, as you'll need to fill them. Keep the "lids" because you'll put them back on.

2. On medium to high heat sauté the onions (finely diced) and the garlic (crushed). Add the rice.
3. Put the removed flesh of the tomatoes in a food processor and then add to the pan along with the sugar and herbs. Add salt and pepper to taste.
4. Preheat the oven at 450 F.
5. When the rice is halfway cooked, remove from the heat. Distribute the filling between the tomatoes in a baking pan. Don't fill them all the way to the top, as the rice will about double in size. Add the lids and sprinkle a good amount of olive oil on each tomato.
6. Optionally add potatoes to the pan, cut in medium pieces. Any leftover filling can also be added between the tomatoes.
7. Add salt, pepper and about ½ cup water.
8. Bake for 45-60 minutes. It's done when the rice is fully cooked.

I hope these new recipes will either inspire you to get in the kitchen and give yourself some well-deserved nutrition and taste or be nice additions to your cooking portfolio if you are already an experienced cook. Being on a weight loss plan is not about denying ourselves the enjoyment of food. On the contrary, you should love yourself enough to want to be kind to you and give you nice and healthy meals to improve your performance. Time spent on taking care of ourselves is never wasted. If you want to take it one step ahead, feel free to try out the new recipes with your loved ones to show them that they too can take steps to improve their own nutrition. If you have children, show them how to cook simple dishes with you and help them prepare for the time when they will have to make their own nutrition choices.

Conclusion

Thank you for making it through to the end of *Intermittent Fasting and Autophagy*. It has indeed been a terrible lot of information you have had to take in, but let's hope you now have the toolkit to use intermittent fasting to your advantage and activate your autophagy to assist in your weight loss goals.

The next step is always more research. If you have spotted some IF protocol you would like to try or if you just want to learn more, you are always welcome to do your own research, find people like you who can give you advice and maybe research on what the specialists have to say. If this process leads you to adopt intermittent fasting,

Finally, if you found this book useful in any way, a review on Amazon is always appreciated! Best of luck in your weight loss endeavors. I hope you always feel healthy, happy and fulfilled and it would be an honor and a pleasure if this book has assisted you in feeling this way. Never forget to love yourself and improve yourself only out of self-love!

Description

When it comes to weight loss and fat loss, most people have a lot of advice to give, with many of them trying to sell you something you don't even need. You may have tried everything and found yourself failing because no matter how expensive it was, it was unsustainable. But why rely on pricey services and products when all you need to lose weight and fat and lead a healthier lifestyle is something you can do completely by yourself? How? Welcome to the world of intermittent fasting. If fasting makes you think of starvation, deprivation and the such, you are not alone. However, this is not at all what it is about.

Fasting has in fact been used forever, not only by people but also by animals in nature. As Hippocrates of Kos first observed, animals when they are sick will most likely not wish to eat, as happens with humans. Fasting has a lot of healing properties for our body, with the most important one being that it activates autophagy, a homeostatic mechanism which is responsible for the destruction of damaged cells and the regeneration of the body. Reports of weight loss with autophagy are very encouraging, as it seems that people who lose fat in this way tend to avoid the loose skin which is otherwise quite usual when someone loses a lot of weight and also get other health benefits.

Activating autophagy is a three-way process. You can use intermittent fasting, a low carb diet, and exercise. This book will walk you through the first one. In these very well researched 9 chapters, you will get to answer many of your questions about intermittent fasting and how to implement it, such as but not limited to:

- Is fasting dangerous? What can it do for me?
- Which intermittent fasting models are there?
- Am I allowed to intermittent fast? Which model is ideal for me?

- How can I activate autophagy and is there too much of a good thing when it comes to it?

Included, tips and tricks for your intermittent fasting endeavors and weight loss in general, a handful of recipes to spice up your meal preps and fill you with nutrients and many more!

So, you shouldn't wait any longer to find out about intermittent fasting and take advantage of the wonderful mechanisms that already are to be found in the human body. The journey to a better performance, a better mood, a better life and a better you has just started!

www.ingramcontent.com/pod-product-compliance
Lightning Source LLC
Chambersburg PA
CBHW072201280526
45788CB00002B/821